INTERMITTENT FASTING

FOR BEGINNERS

Author

Karl Small

Legal & Disclaimer

The information contained in this book and its contents are not designed to replace or take the place of any form of medical or professional advice and are not meant to replace the need for independent medical, financial, legal or other professional advice or services, as may be required. The content and information in this book have been provided for educational and entertainment purposes only.

The content and information contained in this book has been compiled from sources deemed reliable, and it is accurate to the best of the Author's knowledge, information and belief. However, the Author cannot guarantee its accuracy and validity and cannot be held liable for any errors and/or omissions. Furthermore, changes are periodically made to this book as and when needed. Where appropriate and/or necessary, you must consult a professional (including but not limited to your doctor, attorney, financial advisor or such other professional advisor) before using any of the suggested remedies, techniques, or information in this book.

Upon using the contents and information contained in this book, you agree to hold harmless the Author from and against any damages, costs, and expenses, including any legal fees potentially resulting from the application of any of the information provided by this book. This disclaimer applies to any loss, damages or injury caused by the use and application, whether directly or indirectly, of any advice or information presented, whether for breach of contract, tort, negligence, personal injury, criminal intent, or under any other cause of action.

You agree to accept all risks of using the information presented inside this book.

You agree that by continuing to read this book, where appropriate and/or necessary, you shall consult a professional before using any of the suggested remedies, techniques, or information in this book.

Table of Contents

AUTOPHAGY:

Activate Your Natural Self-Cleansing Process to Lose Weight, Reduce Inflammation, Boost Energy and Live Longer Through Intermittent Fasting, Keto Diet, Exercise and Other Methods

By Jaida Ellison

FOREWORD

This book is a full package of everything you need to know about autophagy. It gives very important details about this emerging concept in a casual relaxed tone. The reader grasps life-saving tips and knowledge, without even knowing. The vocabulary and language used are basic and do not require expertise or prior knowledge to understand.

This book enables the reader to understand more about autophagy, its types, mechanisms and how it affects the body (short and long-term benefits), ways of implementing it and most importantly how to live an autophagy-based lifestyle .

This book helps the reader retrace his or her steps, especially as pertains to food (eating *healthy*). Longman dictionary describes food as a material consisting essentially of proteins, carbohydrates and fat that is taken in by living things and supplies energy and sustains processes (e.g. growth as well as repair) necessary for survival. This definition shows how far we have deviated from the principal purpose of eating, considered to be both to nourish and sustain our life. Exercising is not left out. Autophagy basically talks about living healthy.

Each chapter in this book is a gold mine. There is always something new and fascinating, separately conveying and driving home their respective points. Therefore, even if you decide to pick chapters randomly, a lot of knowledge and information will still be gained.

Autophagy is discussed in phases designed progressively to increase assimilation. Firstly, a brief rundown of autophagy is given, followed by more exciting details.

INTRODUCTION

Nowadays, every step taken in our world revolves around technological efficiency. More efficient cars are being built. They are faster, more advanced, and most importantly, they are made to consume less energy (e.g. fuel, diesel, etc.). Today, cars that can use water, electricity and many other cleaner sources of energy are being manufactured and marketed around the globe. This drive for improved efficiency is not limited to cars alone. It applies to almost every other thing (or technology) in the world today. Our bodies are no different. Scientists and researchers, medical practitioners, nutritionists and many more professionals around the world work around the clock to improve the efficiency of the human body. The purpose of their work can be summarized in one sentence: improve the quality of human life, reduce mortality, and increase human longevity.

Living a healthy and fulfilling life doesn't happen by merely wishing it. Without a doubt, some people are naturally stronger than others. For some reason, most likely genetics, their bodies are more robust (able to withstand more). This cannot change the fact that living healthy will prolong the quality of your life. Not just the quality, but its length too.

Over the years, many lifestyles have been adopted to achieve these targets (longevity). Examples include vegan lifestyles, exercise-based living, etc., all with the same intent: to improve the quality of life and increase longevity.

Let's introduce autophagy, shall we! Autophagy can be described as a combination of all these healthy lifestyles. Autophagy refreshes, enhances and boosts the body in a way never before seen. This is a *book of life.* It is bound to affect your life positively. Why? The answer is simple and straightforward.

We all want to live longer! This is something we all want.

To live a life free from sickness, pain and discomfort. Although this book focuses on autophagy, an emerging health concept, it is a must-read for everyone, both young and old. This is not a law book that only educates the reader on the dos and don'ts of autophagy and how to achieve it. It is practically oriented and offers endless resources on the subject. To cap it all, details on autophagy and the ways to achieve it are provided in a completely new way.

Maintaining a healthy lifestyle cannot be overemphasized. Recent statistics have highlighted that disease occurrence is more than ever on the increase (number of people affected by disease). A new case study has shown that over one fifth of the world's population was afflicted by diverse diseases. The most insane thing is the fact that millions of people are diagnosed with diseases every day. Further statistics show that every second, thousands of people are dying from a disease. Astonishingly, scientists predict that these statistics will go up.

What makes autophagy intriguing is the fact that it is rooted in most parts of our everyday lives. This includes how and what we eat, the quantity of food we consume, daily routines, working out and much more. Simply put, living healthy stems from our lifestyle. Unhealthy foods are the cliché while exercising is now seen as a luxury. Although medications, exercise and adequate rest all contribute to a good management and treatment of illnesses, the role of a proper and healthy lifestyle has taken center stage in today's handling of diseases.

A proper diet can tilt you towards living a healthy and enjoyable life as a person. An improper diet would complicate your health, increase suffering and ultimately reduce your quality of life, should it be now or later in the future. You might think about not living a healthy life as digging your own grave. The folly of not living healthy as a person can be compared to pressing a self-destruct button.

Welcome on board! The autophagy flight just took off.

CHAPTER ONE: What is Autophagy?

Did you know the human body is partly cannibalistic by nature?

The body feeds on its unwanted parts. The million-dollar question then is why? Sometimes to achieve our aims or desires we might have to take a step back. Even in construction building, some of the most popular edifices around the world have been adjusted and re-adjusted until the perfect structure was achieved, although in the case of our bodies, consider these adjustments to be constant, as perfection is never really achieved. Autophagy literally means self-eating. It is coined from two words: *auto* (pertaining to self) and *phagy* (eating/devouring).

Autophagy can be defined as the process by which our body reshapes and rebuilds itself, removing unwanted components. It can be defined as the way our body cleans out damaged cells in order to grow new, healthier cells. Autophagy is induced by nutrient limitation and cellular stress, which governs the degradation of the majority of long-lived proteins, protein aggregates and whole organelles. It enables cells to survive stress from both external environment such as nutrient deprivation, as well as internal stress like accumulation of damaged organelles and pathogen invasion.

To put it simply, the body is in search of its masterpiece. Our body pushes itself to the limit, even without our personal effort. It keeps removing unwanted components in a desperate search for non-attainable perfection. On the upside, perfection is very difficult to achieve. Sometimes achieving your own personal best is more than enough.

To highlight the growing effect of autophagy in our world today, the Nobel Assembly at Karolinska Institutet awarded the 2016 Nobel prize in Physiology or Medicine to Yoshinori Ohsumi for his discoveries of the mechanisms of autophagy. Without any doubt, autophagy is not only here to stay, but it is bound to revolutionize medicine altogether.

Basic terminologies

For a better understanding of this book and the brainstorming ideas and principles it embodies, certain terms have to be explained.

Firstly, let's define the term **recycling:** it means to treat or process (used or waste) materials so as to make suitable for reuse: e.g. recycling paper to save trees. Why do we need to recycle? We basically recycle to conserve natural resources, save energy and space. Without recycling there would be heaps of waste everywhere, pollution of the environment and there would be wastage of our limited natural resources.

To recycle means to pass through a series of changes in order to return to a previous stage in a cyclic process. In the context of this book, recycling refers to the way the body degrades cellular components, dead cells, foreign agents, etc. through the aid of lysosomes. Sometimes the degradation process might involve lysing and remodeling. Other times it might just involve lysing, without any remodeling. How does this relate to the human body? For proper functioning, the body must break down damaged or unnecessary organelles and other cellular constituents. Lysosomes are organelles found in the cells of most animal species. They contain digestive enzymes that help to break down biological (related to the body) macromolecules and foreign bodies. You can call them the soldiers of the autophagic process.

Next is the concept of the **cell:** the cell is the building block of the body. In a building it would be a piece of block, in bread making an ounce of flour and in the constitution it would be the individual clauses, etc. Understanding the cell and its activities is the first step required in understanding autophagy.

The idea behind autophagy

Where did the idea come from? Our bodies where the first scientists to implement autophagy. They have been practicing autophagy long before the first scientists got wind of it. Another good question should be: why does the body deliberately initiate autophagy? Well, the answer to that is a funny one. It has no option. They are stuck with each other.

Even growth is an autophagic process. In growing children and young adults, the body is always shaping and remodeling its tissues to fine-tune the growth process. The scientist is simply trying to understand this amazing technology. Yeah! technology gotten from the body. This should not be surprising, as many ideas behind some of the most groundbreaking discoveries came from natural processes.

Types of autophagy

Cells have two important protein degradation pathways. They are the Ubiquitin Proteasome System (UPS) and the Autophagy-Lysosome Pathway (ALP). The UPS, which is the body's major proteolytic pathway degrades short-lived, soluble proteins while the Autophagy Lysosome Pathway is responsible for degrading or lying older cytoplasmic proteins, soluble and insoluble misfolded proteins, and body organelles. This book is more interested in this second pathway: the **Autophagic Lysosomes Pathway.**

There are three major types of autophagy: **macro-autophagy, micro autophagy and chaperone autophagy** . All three types require certain enzymes and genes to function.

1. **Macro-autophagy** is one the most important types of autophagy. Its activities are carried out in many parts of the cell. Macro-autophagy is divided in two: the bulk and the selective. Selective macro-autophagy is divided into subtypes. These subtypes are named according to the parts of the cell they target. They are lipophagy (degradation of the lipid part of the cell), pexophagy (degradation of cellular peroxisomes), chlorophagy (degradation of cellular chlorophyll), autophagy (degradation of the mitochondria) and ribophagy (degradation of ribosomes). Other subtypes are emerging, as research on autophagy is still ongoing. In essence, macroautophagy is concerned with degrading (removing) damaged cell organelles from the cell.

2. **Micro-autophagy** is more specialized. It involves the direct engulfment of selected materials. This could be foreign bodies such as materials, bacteria, or any element foreign to the body.

3. **Chaperone autophagy** is the most complex type of autophagy. For chaperone autophagy to take place, a certain protein known as the hsc70 complex must be present. For degradation (lysis) to occur, the particle to be degraded must contain a recognition site for this complex. Binding then occurs at this degradation site (between the recognition site and the hsc70

complex). Chaperone autophagy is the most selective form of autophagy. It screens materials before sending them past the lysosomal barrier.

Why is autophagy activated?

Autophagy is the body's way of responding to stress and physiological conditions. This is an important point to note because it embodies the whole autophagic process, which is the fact that autophagy is always induced. It never occurs on its own, there is always a reason for it. Examples of inducing factors include food deprivation, hyperthermia and hypoxia.

The mechanisms behind autophagy

The autophagic process is a very complex one. However, it was simplified and explained in the most elementary form here. It begins with the formation of a membrane vesicle (usually double stranded). This membrane vesicle then forms a cover around the cell's cytoplasm, altered proteins, old proteins (proteins that have stayed in the cell for a long time) and organelles. It then fuses with autophagic soldiers (lysosomes). The formation of the double-membrane proteins is one of the most important steps in cellular autophagy.

The entire process is regulated by proteins known as "tag proteins". Below are some important autophagic regulators.

Autophagy in steps (autophagic process)

Some of the term descriptions are pretty advanced. However, understanding them would help you grasp autophagy better. The terms were simplified as much as possible.

1. Sequestration

This is the first step in the autophagy process. During this stage, two membranes expand and cover the cytoplasm. These membranes are known as phagophores. The phagophore does not only enclose the cytoplasm. It equally encloses the organelles within it. The purpose of enclosing them (cytoplasm and organelles) is to prepare them for degradation. Before the end of this stage, the phagophore becomes an organelle called the autophagosome.

2. Transportation

Earlier in the book when we discussed terminologies, we described lysosomes as autophagic soldiers. That rank was well deserved, as the whole autophagic process revolves around them. For degradation to occur, the autophagosome has to connect with the lysosome. Essentially, the transportation stage (step 2) involves the formation of structures that will aid the transfer of materials from the autophagosome to the lysosome.

In order to connect with the lysosomes, the autophagosome fuses with an intermediate organelle called the endosome. Together, they form what is called an amphisome. The amphisome can readily fuse with the lysosomes.

3. Lysing/degradation

This is the final step in the autophagy process. The amphisome fuses with the lysosome, conveying its contents. The lysosome then releases enzymes known as hydrolases. They lyse (degrade) all the materials conveyed from the amphisome. The resulting structure, which now consists of degraded cellular material, is now called an autolysosome. The degraded products (amino acids) are now transported from the autolysosome into the cellular fluid. They are either marked for excretion or can be used to build new cells.

Autophagic regulators

-Insulin/IGF-1

Although Atg proteins are the major regulators in the autophagic process, the insulin/IGF-1 pathway plays a vital role. The pathway promotes growth, morphogenesis and survival.

Nutrient deprivation also plays a role in autophagy. The body tries to generate nutrients for itself. It does this by lysing (degrading) old and worn out cells and using them as a nutrient source. To carry this out, an Atg protein is hyper-phosphorylated by TORC1.

Apart from its role in nutrient generation (autophagic pathway), TORC1 equally contributes to the activation of several factors that oversee transcription or translation of some proteins by phosphorylation. Some of these proteins are needed (utilized) in the autophagic pathway. TOR regulates the induction of autophagy. It does this alongside protein kinase A and SCh9.

-DRAM and p53

The p53 suppressor is found in about half of the human population. It exists in a mutated form and helps to induce autophagy. It is equally important in helping the body to carry out apoptosis. Apoptosis simply means programmed cell death.

-FOXO and ROS

Recent research has shown that FOXO aids in the transcription of autophagy related genes. Some of these genes include Atg8/LC3, Atg12, Vps34, and Atg6. In muscles undergoing atrophy, Atg6 induces protein degradation in the atrophied cells.

ROS (Reactive Oxygen Species) have been found to play a role in starvation induced autophagy. During starvation, the body degrades (breaks down) old cells. Some of the nutrients from these degraded cells are then moved to more important cells. You can compare this to a generator powering a whole building. In a situation where the fuel tank has very little fuel left in it, a compromise has to be reached. The generator operator would have to reduce the load. Unimportant devices are turned off, while the important devices are kept running.

CHAPTER TWO: How to Achieve Autophagy

Boosting autophagy in your body simply means trying to make your body operate at its optimum. You are maximizing your output and increasing your body's efficiency. Amazingly, not only is your body operating at its maximum, but it is operating on **clean energy.** You can call this the body's version of green energy. You are supplying your body with nutrients and energy in the cleanest (healthiest) way possible.

There are three major ways to boost autophagy in the body.

Keto diet

This is a simple and natural way of activating autophagy without forgoing some of your favorite meals. The idea is to reduce carbohydrate levels. When carbohydrate levels are low, the body has no choice but to use fat as a fuel source. This is the concept behind the extremely popular ketogenic diet.

Keto diets are diets high in fat and low in carbohydrates (e.g. teak, bacon and peanut butter shakes). Between 60 and 70 percent of your overall calories come from fat. Proteins are the next major contributors. They make up about 20 to 30% of the body's calories.

Protein provides 20 to 30 percent of calories, while only 5 percent comes from carbs. This shows that carbohydrates are the most insignificant part of our diet. While proteins can be converted into sugar (in the absence of carbohydrates), fats cannot.

So basically, in ketosis you lose excess body fat while retaining muscle. Ketogenesis equally aids the body in resolving cancerous tumors, lowers the risk of diabetes and protects the body from brain disorders such as epilepsy. Ketosis can be said to be an autophagy hack. Through keto-diets you can gain the benefits of autophagy, without stressing your body too much. In keto-diets there is a gradual shift from burning carbs (glucose) to ketones. Autophagy is keto-based, hence very little carb is involved in autophagy.

Fasting

-Water Fasting

Water fasting is a milder form of fasting. Fasting (in all forms) is one of the most effective ways of achieving autophagy. An individual undergoing a water fast can drink water. Although he or she will not consume anything else except water for twenty-four hours, water fasts might not be as effective as a full fast. A full fast does not involve water. Nothing is eaten within twenty-four hours. Water fasting benefits include weight loss, body cleansing, cellular regeneration and, most importantly, autophagy. It is increasing in popularity.

Also, the presence of oxygen in the water helps the body. It assists the body in eliminating harmful toxins. That is why water fasting is nicknamed the expert cleanser. Whenever water and fasting meet, detoxification must occur.

Water is calorie-free. That is why water enhances metabolism and ketogenesis. There are links between drinking water and weight loss. As the body shifts to ketosis during water fasting, it can use up excess fat. Water fasting also boosts the body's healing process. It reduces inflammation in the body and lowers blood sugar levels while enhancing the activities of the heart and brain. Additionally, drinking water supports collagen synthesis in the skin.

Tips (on water fasting)

Fasting requires a lot of effort. Before you begin a water fast, you need to prepare yourself mentally. You need to always picture the light at the end of the tunnel. Visualizing your goals will help motivate you.

Before commencing your water fast, you should have a doctor's consultation to decide the duration of your program.

Abstaining from food for a week and taking nothing but water can be very tough especially at the beginning. You might feel hungry or weak as your body will be in a state of ketosis after 3-4 days. The body adapts to this 'new' system and the fasting process becomes much easier.

Setting the duration of your fast

Fasting essentially means abstinence from all foods. In Islam or Christianity for example, fasting dates are based for days of the week, months or a year. It can be done for different durations.

Water fasting can last for as little as 3 days to a whole month based on the objective and capability of the person. For example, it is suggested that individuals suffering from chronic illnesses should avoid water fasts longer than 3 days.

The amount of water taken in a day is directly related to the individual's level of activity. Although the amount of water taken in is not critical (in respect to results), most people, irrespective of the amount of water they drink, experience tremendous changes (weight loss, detoxification, autophagy, etc.).

-Skipping meals/intermittent fasting

Skipping meals is another method you can use to achieve autophagy. Unlike ketosis, this method is stressful. At first you might not understand the benefits, but you are bound to become addicted once you start seeing the results. Recent studies have shown that periodic fasting and autophagy can make cancer treatments more productive. Normal body cells are not affected unlike in normal cancer therapy. Modern cancer therapies are very harsh. They make wholesale changes to your body size (weight) and can even affect your looks.

Recent research has shown that intermittent fasting improves brain function, brain structure and neuroplasticity. It helps the brain to reorganize and replenish itself. It equally helps to improve cognitive function and structures.

Intermittent fasting is simply taking skipping meals to another level. Intermittent fasting should be adopted to suit your capabilities and personal targets. Whichever way you choose to practice it, you are bound to reap some amazing benefits. Some of these benefits include increased resistance to diseases and infection, reduced body weight, increased lifespan, improved cardiovascular function, increased brain function and a whole lot more.

Children, pregnant women, people with ulcers, low sugar levels and persons with food associated ailments (diseases) are advised to practice intermittent fasting mildly. In some cases, they should avoid it totally, most especially pregnant women.

So then, the question is:*How can intermittent fasting improve autophagy?* Well let's compare this to a packed fridge. This fridge belongs to Mr. Food (hypothetic). He keeps packing his fridge with food. The fridge is now in layers (layers of food). Some of these foods reach their expiry dates. Mr. Food can't see or notice this. Naturally, decomposition begins, followed by a foul odor. Cool story, right?

This mirrors what happens in our bodies when we keep over feeding. The body is packed up with digestion products (glucose, fat, amino acids) that keep piling up. There's a popular adage: " **too much of anything is never good".** This is a universal truth. Our bodies, the atmosphere, water, soil, etc., all exist on a delicate balance. Nature finds a way to balance itself. No excesses, just perfection!

Intermittent fasting is one of the ways we can help our body to achieve this balance. Fasting forces the body to use up its stores. Some cells die during this process (autophagy). These cells are replaced by the body when you feed again. *Hence, the body is renewed and refreshed!*

-Longer fasts (no food or water)

Intermittent fasting is a vital tool for improving health, achieving weight loss, detoxification, cellular regeneration and autophagy. There is enough evidence to back this up. However, longer fasts have proven to be more effective. *Please, always fast according to your capabilities. You can achieve similar results with both water fasts, intermittent fasts and full fasts.*

Full fasting can take many forms. The most drastic is a "dry fast", which entails avoiding all edibles and fluids (food or water). **Never start a full fast without consulting a medical practitioner.** Full fasts can be very severe and shouldn't be done for more than 48 hours.

Long fasts and autophagy

The most outstanding benefit of full fasts is their ability to induce autophagy. If you abstain from food, your body will be forced to use up its stores. Old cells are recycled as well. They are used to build new cells (autophagy). After 24 hours, the body uses up most of the glycogen in the liver.

In respect to weight loss, the body loses around 1-2 pounds a day. This happens because it is shedding water weight and protein. However, the body's dependence on protein as a source of energy is short-lived. Using protein would mean breaking down muscles, some of which might be essential/delicate.

This makes fat a more reliable/suitable energy source. Hence, after a few days, the body switches to its fat stores for energy (ketosis). Fat is more energy-dense per pound than protein, so weight loss in this phase is slower. It reduces to just over 1 pound every 2 days.

A long fast is the easiest way of staying in ketosis for an extended duration. It forces the body to rely completely on its own fat stores instead of dietary fat. Being in ketosis makes weight loss easy. Ketosis helps suppress hunger (especially after the first few days, which are usually tough). Fasting also enables you to totally get your mind off food. It saves you the stress of thinking about what to eat next and bothering on the amount of food you are eating.

Full fast is an effective means to lose a lot of weight quickly. However, many people begin to gain it all back again because they just go back to their old eating pattern.

Like most "crash diets," fasting will help you lose weight, but won't help you maintain the status quo, unless you also make permanent changes in your diet after the fast is over.

As we noted earlier, long fasts promote autophagy, which can be compared to "spring cleaning" for your cells. Since the body is basically eating itself, it has a chance to eliminate any junk or waste products that may have built up, and repair the harm caused by oxidative stress. This is one of the substantial benefits of fasting even for people who have a healthy weight. Autophagy also has powerful anti-aging and muscle-building properties.

Recent research has shown that an extended fast (10 days on average) was beneficial to people suffering from hypertension, also noting that even though the patients didn't start the fasting program to lose weight, all of them had an average weight loss of around 15 pounds. Full fasts (up to 5 days) may also have some benefits for chemotherapy patients.

Another effect of full fasts is mental clarity. It is a way to break free from overeating patterns or other food disorders. Fasting is practiced by many religious groups because it enhances meditation and mindfulness. Briefly put, fasting declogs the mind and increases focus.

Exercise

Working out stresses the muscles (damages them in a good way). The muscles are torn and rebuilt. This makes them stronger and more resistant. Increasing your muscular strength improves your body's condition. People who exercise regularly are less prone to diseases and infections. Researchers have discovered that exercise improves the human immune system. Resistance training is usually the most effective type of exercise, not just for autophagy, but the body as a whole. When done at intervals, the body's conditioning improves. You tear up your muscles, rebuild stronger ones and stimulate autophagy.

Exercise is in essence a physical method of achieving autophagy. You use up your body stores directly when you exercise. Most people describe exercise as refreshing. Well, that is not just a feeling. It is actually happening. *Exercise catalyzes regeneration* (development of new cells). To regenerate means to replace lost or damaged tissue. So not only are new cells being produced, old ones are encouraged to die.

Exercising is very important in the treatment of any disease. How rigorous the exercise is, depends on your doctor's approval. Exercise improves your body's use of insulin and may lower blood sugar levels apart from helping to use up some of the excess glucose. Exercise equally helps to increase blood circulation, enhance kidney function, reduce risk of developing diabetes and in general helps to improve the body's condition.

Exercise can equally lower the chance of having a heart attack or stroke and can improve circulation. Furthermore, it has been proven that exercise benefits the brain greatly. It increases blood circulation to the brain and helps increase the brain's efficiency. Exercise is highly recommended, especially for those who are obese/overweight. Care should be taken not to over work the body in one go. Exercise should be gradual and progressive. A minimum of 150 minutes a week (total exercise time) is recommended.

A large number of diseases target and attack the muscles. They reduce their mass, finally rendering them useless. The body cannot function without strong muscles. Exercising daily helps your body keep its muscles alive and strong.

You do not have to follow a drastic, severe exercising program. All you have to do is try to exercise at least three hours a week. Walking in a park for an hour, running on a treadmill, going to the mall for three hours, in other words simply walking around often is a good start to keep your body in shape. When you go shopping, try to park far from the entrance so you have to walk more on your way there and back.

Exercising helps your blood circulate through your body and helps your body burn fat and bad calories. By exercising, the sugar in your blood is used to help your muscles function and therefore not be stagnant in your organs and arteries. It is a simple process: more you eat, more you need to exercise and more you exercise, more you need to eat.

According to doctors and researchers, exercising is the best way to fight disease. However, it does so with a daily routine or at least a tri-weekly habit. Just walking around the block once a month is not enough, extra effort is needed.

Exercising helps you feel better about yourself as it releases endorphins in your body, the same endorphins you would get by eating your favorite food. Working out fights the high level of cholesterol and keeps cholesterol related diseases away.

If you plan on exercising daily and at a high level, talk about it with your doctor. He will help you find the best program for your needs and physical and medical abilities. You will have to take it slowly, step by step. Do not try to run a marathon on the first day or go on a five-mile run because you want to burn the calories. You will burn as many calories walking a mile at a good pace as you would by running the same distance.

Dietary tips

To achieve autophagy, you can try some of these dietary tips. At least once or twice a week, you should limit your protein intake to 15-25 grams a day. This gives the body nearly a day to recycle stored proteins, reduce inflammation and cleanse body cells. The best part is that the muscle mass remains the same. It does not shrink or reduce. During this abstinence period (food abstinence), the body is forced to consume its stored proteins and toxins. Skipping breakfast (say twice a week), helps to promote autophagy in the body. It gives the body time to clean itself (eliminate lingering toxins).

Research has shown that about 30% of women respond to intermittent fasting more severely. To curb these effects, a fat-based breakfast is recommended. Basically, you are required to keep carbohydrates and fat from your meals (for a whole day). However, the quantity taken should be regulated. Fats are energy Kings. Half of kilogram of fat gives three or four times more energy than proteins or carbohydrates of the same quantity. So, taking in a very small quantity of fat is usually more than enough. This way, you are not starving your body, while promoting autophagy.

Your daily meals have a direct effect on your body. Some foods, when consumed in large quantities are unhealthy, while others have minimal or no negative effects on the body. Therefore, managing what you eat, knowing the calorie content, the ingredients and how they affect your body is very important. Generally, three major classes of food appear in most of our meals or diets. They include carbohydrates, fats and proteins. Vegetables, fruits and fiber appear much less in meals and diets. To influence your health positively, an understanding of these food classes and their effects on the body is very important.

Carbohydrates

These are one of the most popular food classes. They exist as starches, sugar and fiber in foods such as grains, fruits, vegetables, milk products and sweets. They increase blood sugar levels and affect the body more than any other food. Therefore, knowing what foods contain carbohydrates and regulating the amount per meal is helpful for blood glucose control. Carbohydrates in your meal should come from healthy sources like vegetables, fruits, whole grains and legumes. Also, carbohydrates coming from whole grain (high fibers) are recommended. Those originating from sources with added sugars, fats and salt should be avoided.

Carbohydrate control and regulation is the bedrock to achieving autophagy. Eating carbohydrates is not bad (unhealthy) in essence. The quantity simply has to be reduced, and carbohydrates from healthier sources should be integrated into meal plans. Eating carbohydrates from healthy sources can equally help you to lose excess body weight and generally make you healthier.

Proteins

Proteins are an important part of our diet. In an experiment where an individual consumed a given quantity of protein and another consumed the same quantity of carbohydrates, the individual who took the carbohydrates was most likely to be hungry first. This shows how important proteins are in helping create satiety. Proteins mildly contribute to the glucose (sugar levels) in the body and are usually increased in most recommended meal plans (health meal plans). However, to achieve autophagy, proteins are not needed in high quantities. Proteins are equally the building blocks of the body, and generally help the body to recover from stress and ailments.

Fats

These are the number one energy givers in the body. Fats are an important component in the creation of balanced diets, and more importantly, in achieving autophagy. When digested, fats undergo ketosis (an important energy cycle the body experiences in times of starvation). Therefore, when you take the right amount of fats, you can induce artificial starvation. Most especially healthy fats are from fish (e.g. trout and salmon), nuts, seeds, olive oil, canola oil, other vegetable oils, avocado, and soft margarine. Fats don't raise blood glucose but are high in calories. Their high calorie content and energy giving ability means that very small quantities can sustain the body. Health wise, it is advisable to use non-saturated fatty acids as against saturated fatty acids. Sources of saturated fatty acids include butter, red meat, cakes, pastries and deep-fried foods. Instead, plant-based protein and lower fat dairy products should be used more often.

Generally, to create an autophagy inducing diet, fats should be included more in the diet, albeit in differing quantities.

Vegetables and fruit

Vegetables and fruits are beneficial to the body. They help in flushing and cleansing the body. They contain many vitamins and minerals to help supply vital nutrients and regulate vital body activities. They can equally be used as snacks, because most of them contain fibers. Hence, they can easily cause satiety. Fruits also contain natural sugars which are less harmful to the body.

Other methods to induce autophagy

-Drugs

Although the use of drugs to achieve autophagy is still relatively untested (in its infancy), certain drugs have the ability to induce autophagy. Although their actions are usually specific (inducing their effects in certain parts of the body), their actions are not generalized.

For example, latrepirdine, resveratrol and lithium are used to stimulate autophagy in patients with Huntington's disease. Since research is presently ongoing, their usage is still very limited.

In the treatment of Alzheimer's disease, certain drugs/substances such as nicotinamide, hydroxy chloroquine, resveratrol, nilotinib, lithium, latrepirdine, metformin, valproic acid and statins have been credited with inducing different levels of autophagy. Equally, in the treatment of Parkinson's disease nilotinib and statins have been credited with inducing autophagy. Lastly, lithium, tamoxifen, and valproic are said to be capable of inducing Amyotrophic lateral sclerosis (ALS).

Most of these drugs are relatively untested. However, advancements are being made as we speak. Their usage is currently limited to neurodegenerative and auto-immune diseases. In the future, it is hoped that autophagy would be more widely used.

-Regulating sleep

It is recommended that we get at least 7-9 hours of sleep a day. Despite these recommendations, modern research has shown that the amount of sleep an individual requires depends on his or her sleep personality. This factor is scientifically called the sleep chronotype. Studies have shown that about 4 sleep personalities exist. Each sleep personality requires a certain amount of sleep a day (different sleep combinations). Certain individuals (based on their sleep personality) can cope with less sleep, while others require more. Sleep plays an important role in body recovery (regeneration of cells). Therefore, knowing the exact amount of sleep you need per day is very important. However, it should be noted that sleep is qualitative and not quantitative. Sleeping for hours under duress and in uncomfortable conditions might not be beneficial for the body. Less hours of sleep in a comfortable and relaxed environment, position or place might be worth more.

-Drink coffee

Modern research has shown that caffeine can induce autophagy in the muscle tissue, liver and heart. Even when taken on a full stomach or with other foods, its ability to induce autophagy is not reduced.

-Turmeric

Turmeric has proven to be effective in inducing autophagy in the cell, specifically in the mitochondria. This is majorly due to curcumin, a nutrient found in turmeric.

-Virgin olive oil

Virgin olive oil contains an antioxidant called oleuropein. Oleuropein is said to have anti-cancerous properties, one of which stems from its ability to induce autophagy.

-Ginger

Ginger consumption can help induce autophagy. This is because ginger contains an active component called 6-shogaol. 6-shogaol has become renowned for its efficiency in the treatment of lung cancer.

-Green Tea

The ingredient responsible for the autophagic ability of green tea is called polyphenol. It is found in both green and white tea. It is organ-specific, with most of its actions focused on the liver, where it helps to prevent inflammation, cancer and liver damage.

-Coconut Oil

Coconut oil is rich in ketones. Ketones are natural components produced by the body in times of starvation. Hence, by taking coconut oil, you are inducing starvation (a fake one) in the body.

-Reishi Mushroom

Even before its autophagy inducing properties where discovered, Reishi mushrooms where used in traditional medicine for decades in Asia. Modern research has shown that Reishi mushrooms can induce autophagy, which in turn produces anticancer effects in those who suffer from breast cancer.

-Vitamin D

Also known as the sunshine vitamin, vitamin D is synthesized naturally in the body (specifically in the skin). Its precursors are activated by sunlight. Those staying in regions where sunlight is minimal or non-existent (e.g. artic regions) might have to take synthesized vitamin D.

Vitamin D is capable of inducing autophagy in the pancreatic islets. Predictably, this will increase insulin production in the pancreas and is therefore very effective in the treatment of type 2 diabetes.

-Melatonin

Melatonin is the only hormone on this list. It plays an important role in the regulation of our circadian rhythm (circadian rhythm is very important in coordinating sleep). Recent studies have shown that melatonin supplementation can induce autophagy in the brain. It helps to protect the brain from cell injury. Cellular injury is one of the leading causes of neuropsychiatric conditions around the world.

-Ginseng (ginseng root)

Ginseng is one of the most important natural supplements in the world today. It is sold around the globe and is even capable of boosting the human immune system. Apart from its immune boosting ability, it also induces autophagy and helps prevent cancer.

CHAPTER THREE

Autophagy in weight loss

Autophagy benefits the body, whether you are overweight or not. However, we will first analyze its use in the treatment of excess body weight.

Excess body weight has been associated with the development of many diseases in the world today. If finding the cause of diseases (a random pick) was tried in a court of law, excess body weight would be incriminated, probably with countless charges. The role it plays in the development of diseases cannot be overstated.

For starters, when is a person said to be overweight? An overweight person is described as heavier than what is generally considered healthy for a given body type and height. Most people don't even know if they are overweight.

How to know if you are overweight:

If in advanced cases an obese individual can easily be assessed visually, this might prove to be difficult in individuals who are only slightly overweight or obese. There are two recommended methods to check this: by referring to the body mass index method and by measuring the waste size.

-Body Mass Index Method

This method measures the weight of a person in relation to his or her height. A score is obtained from the calculation, which is then used to categorize the individual. Normal weight individuals usually fall into a body mass index of about 18.5 to 24.9, while overweight individuals usually fall into a body mass index of about 25.0 and above.

-Waist size

This is another method used in checking the body weight statistics of a person. Overall, having too much fat around the waistline is very unhealthy. For women, having a waist size of more than 35 inches is seen as unhealthy while for men anything more than a waist size of 40 is seen as inappropriate.

Autophagy and excess body weight

What's the secret behind losing weight? Some would say exercise, others might say dieting, while others still might recommend a product (slimming teas, fat burning creams, etc.). The truth is that you cannot lose weight effectively without discipline, which is why stimulating autophagy is the best way to lose weight. Why is this? Because autophagy is the definition of discipline (in terms of health). Autophagy is a combination of dieting, exercising and every other healthy way of losing fat.

There is no need to sugar-coat things. If you do not have a reasonable amount of self-discipline, you might never achieve autophagy effectively.

How it works

Autophagy simply means cell eating. This definition is shorter than the one given in the beginning of the book but is nevertheless a good one.

Autophagy cleans up the body. We previously told a short fictional story about Mr. Food. He packed his fridge with food, some of which was perishable. Even when the fridge got full, he kept adding. The fridge was full to the brim. Some of the items started decomposing, and as expected, the fridge developed a bad smell. Mr. Food didn't stop though. He kept adding more and more food because he loved it too much to let go.

This story might sound funny or ridiculous, but it really describes the way most people treat their body. They keep on packing it with unwanted materials (food). You gain weight when your body builds its muscles. However, when food is in excess, especially for people who live a sedentary type of life, the body begins to deposit these excesses in body tissues, organs and the muscles. The result is an increase in weight (overweight/obese).

Autophagy excels when the body is put to stress. The word stress should not scare you. It just involves living a disciplined and healthy life. You can achieve weight loss through autophagy by following the steps listed in 'how to achieve autophagy'.

And in normal individuals?

It would be a huge mistake to exclude yourself from the recommended steps because you are not overweight. The body always has excesses to burn.

Autophagy in Metabolic Diseases

To a large extent, autophagy borders on what we eat. It is therefore not surprising that it plays a huge role in the body's defense against metabolic diseases.

Metabolic diseases are those diseases that are affected or related to the body's digestion of food. Diabetes is the most popular metabolic disease. *Advancements in autophagy research has been giving more insight into treatment of the disease.*

To understand the role autophagy plays in modern treatment of diabetes, we would have to first understand diabetes (analyze the disease).

Before we move on to how autophagy aids in the treatment of diabetes, we will take a brief look at the symptoms of the disease. Symptom detection has become very important in our world today. *Early detection of any symptom could be the sharp line between life and death.* Nowadays, diabetes is one of the most widespread diseases in the world.

Diagnosis of any medical condition is usually achieved in two ways. One is by observing the characteristic symptoms of the disease. That is to say every disease has its characteristic symptoms or conditions. The second way is through clinical diagnosis. This involves carrying out certain tests on the selected individual.

Diagnosis Using Symptoms

Type 1 and type 2 diabetes share common symptoms. First among them is:

-Weakness/Tiredness/Hunger

Diabetes messes up with the body's energy metabolism. When insulin is not produced in the required quantity, glucose is not properly transported to the body's organs, cells and muscles. *Autophagy reduces this dependence on glucose. An autophagy diet supplies the body with essential nutrients and energy.*

Earlier in the book, we stated how important nutrients are to the body. Diabetes patients will experience weakness due to lack of energy. This weakness is due to an imbalance in the body's energy mechanism. *Autophagy helps correct this!* Tiredness and hunger can equally result from lack of or reduced energy in a diabetic.

-Frequent Urination and Increased Thirst

Like every symptom of diabetes, these symptoms are also linked to glucose metabolism (breakdown). In this case, excess glucose is transported to the kidney as a result of glucose under-utilization. The kidney would normally absorb some of this glucose, but in this case the quantity to be absorbed makes it impossible. Hence, the kidney transports (sends) a part of the excess glucose (that could not be absorbed) into the urine. This process occurs quite often, which causes the frequent urination.

Autophagy reduces the body's dependence on glucose. It creates healthier energy pathways, which prevent all that was listed above. The kidneys have less glucose to process/absorb, consequently reducing the quantity of urine released.

Like all bodily fluids, urine contains water. As a result, frequent urination will lead to dehydration, which is signaled by its own specific symptoms. Thirst is one of the most frequent symptoms that occur in diabetes. And like always, one thing leads to another. Thirst would cause the affected individual to drink more water. In return, drinking more water will lead to increased urine output (frequent urination). Other symptoms such as dryness of the skin, dizziness and tiredness might be experienced as well.

-Dehydration Symptoms

As explained earlier, dehydration is a condition that results from frequent urination caused by diabetes. In more severe cases, other symptoms of dehydration will become more pronounced. These include dizziness, dryness of the skin, itchy skin, dryness of the mouth, blurred vision (result of the changing fluids in the eyes, specifically the retina) and many more.

-Yeast Infections

People suffering from type 2 diabetes are prone to yeast infections. Glucose (sugar) is a natural substrate for yeast. Therefore, the overabundance of glucose that occurs in diabetes promotes the growth of yeast, and invariably yeast infections. (*Autophagy helps to reduce the body's dependence on glucose - reduced blood sugar levels*). Yeast infections are known to grow in the moist parts of the body. This includes between the fingers and sometimes around the pubic region area and under the breasts.

-Difficulty for Wounds to Heal

High blood sugar levels affect the blood's ability to clot and coagulate (hinders the blood clotting pathway).

-Sharp Loss in Weight

Following damage to the pancreas and the resulting reduction in body glucose levels, the body has to find an alternative source of energy to carry out its numerous activities. It turns to its fatty stores (muscles around the body) and breaks them down, thus creating a new pathway for energy. Continuous breakdown in body fat leads to loss of weight. This process occurs quite quickly which brings about the sharp loss in weight. *Autophagy ensures the body's fatty stores are replenished. It balances the body's energy mechanism and increases overall efficiency.*

Classical Symptoms of Gestational Diabetes

The symptoms occurring in gestational diabetes are not exclusive to it. They also include normal diabetes symptoms such as thirst, frequent urination, tiredness/weakness and sometimes loss of weight.

The metabolic syndrome and CHD

The first abnormality in type 2 diabetes is insulin resistance. It is found in people even before diabetes can be diagnosed. It simply means that your body becomes resistant to the effects of insulin and finds it increasingly difficult over time to keep your blood sugar down to a normal level. When insulin resistance is found in combination with other risk factors, it is called metabolic syndrome (the same combination used to be known as insulin resistance syndrome). About 1 in 4 adults in the UK has metabolic syndrome, and while not all of them have diabetes now, many or even most of them will go on to develop it unless they do some serious work to improve their lifestyle (adopting healthier and more productive living patterns - Autophagic lifestyle).

The International Diabetes Federation has come up with a definition of the metabolic syndrome that involves having at least three of the risk factors listed in the book. Each of them on their own increases the risk of CHD. Add them together, and they more than triple your risk of CHD compared to someone who doesn't have them.

Diabetes and autophagy

Autophagy plays an important role in regulating the activities of the pancreatic islets. It helps to stimulate insulin secretion, especially in times of crisis (low insulin levels). Insulin helps to balance glucose levels in the body.

Not only does autophagy stimulate insulin secretion, it equally helps to protects the pancreatic islets from oxidative stress. In-vitro and in-vivo studies (inside and outside the body) have also shown that autophagy plays a role in their function and survival (pancreatic islets).

Autophagy counters the destructive effects of apoptosis. Apoptosis means programmed cell death. Just like autophagy, apoptosis is a naturally occurring process in the body. However, apoptosis can be mis-controlled, leading to the destruction of body cells that where not marked for destruction.

CHAPTER FOUR: Autophagy in Neurodegenerative Disorders

Medical and scientific research has shown that *neuronal autophagy* plays a critical role in maintaining the body's cellular activities. It plays an equally important role in maintaining nervous system health. Autophagy clears up aggregated proteins. Many scientists believe that these aggregated proteins are behind the development of many neurodegenerative diseases.

In past times, it was believed that neuronal autophagy had little or no effects on the development of neurodegenerative diseases. However, recent studies have revealed the importance of autophagy in non-proliferating cells, particularly in body neurons.

Autophagy plays a vital role in neuroprotection , by implementing multiple key molecular regulations of autophagy pathway. Autophagy helps revive the body's cells, especially those under stress. Autophagy equally aids in the maintenance of cellular homeostasis. Increasing evidence indicates that autophagy machineries are derailed in diverse human diseases, including most neurodegenerative disorders, cancers and inflammatory disorders. Derailed autophagy contributes to neuron degeneration and neuronal cell death disease pathology.

Plenty of evidence has shown the importance of autophagy in the regulation of neurodegenerative disorders. A better understanding of neuronal autophagy will ultimately help medical practitioners develop potential therapeutic interventions targeting autophagic dysregulation.

A part of these neurodegenerative disorders will be discussed below, along with the contributions of autophagy to their treatment.

Parkinson's disease

This is a neurodegenerative disease. Autophagy plays a huge role in the regulation of these diseases. Parkinson's disease is a progressive nervous system disease that affects movement. Symptoms have a slow onset, usually with a barely noticeable tremor in one part of the body, generally the hands. Although tremors are the most popular symptom, other symptoms such as stiffness or slowing of movement might be found.

In the initial stages of Parkinson's disease, the face becomes nearly expressionless. Arms become stiff and movement becomes almost robotic. Speech becomes incoherent and unclear. The disease worsens with time.

Currently, Parkinson's disease is incurable, and medications are palliative. In more complex forms of the disease, surgery might be required to reduce its effects.

Symptoms

As previously stated, any discussion on a disease without proper analysis of the symptoms is incomplete. Early detection of a disease's symptoms would most likely make treatment more effective.

Signs and symptoms of Parkinson's disease are not consistent. Early (mild) signs usually go unnoticed. Most of the time, symptoms begin on one side of the body, and they usually remain worse on that side as the condition progresses

Frequently encountered symptoms:

- *Tremor*

Tremors usually begin in the extremities. The most popular is rubbing of the thumb and forefinger back-and-forth. This is known as a pill-rolling tremor. Tremors might continue even when the body is at rest. Parkinson's disease slows down movements, making easy actions look very complex.

Movement becomes restricted, and some patients might need assistance or a walking stick.

-*Rigid muscles*

Muscles become very rigid and stiff.

-Impaired posture and balance

Posture becomes irregular, patients appear to bend, walk irregularly or without balance.

-Poor reflexes

Reflex actions become more difficult. Patients can even find it difficult to blink.

-Speech changes

Patients' tone of voice becomes soft and irregular. Sometimes the voice might be altered completely.

-Difficulty in writing

Writing becomes very difficult or nearly impossible.

-Presence of Lewy bodies

This symptom can't be seen with the naked eye. It requires a clinical test, after which it is analyzed by medical personnel.

Lewy bodies are important in the diagnosis of Parkinson's disease, and their appearance is almost confirmatory of the presence of the disease.

If you have any of the above symptoms, seek medical advice/assistance.

Causes

Parkinson's disease results from the destruction of the brain's nerve cells. Almost all symptoms have nervous links or origins. Attack on the nerve cells usually affects dopamine levels (dopamine is a neurotransmitter associated with the feeling of pleasure). It is usually this decrease in dopamine levels that causes the symptoms.

Parkinson's disease is currently incurable! We will soon discuss the role autophagy plays in its treatment.

Parkinson's disease and autophagy

Researchers believe that regular exercise (anaerobic exercise) and caffeine consumption can help reduce chances of developing the disease. It is not surprising that both of them promote autophagy.

Some of the pathologies associated with Parkinson's disease (PD) are oxidative stress, mitochondrial dysfunction and protein aggregation. They are all linked with autophagy. Autophagy had previously been regarded as a nutrient based body response. However, increasing recent research has shown that basal and constitutive autophagy is needed for neuronal survival and that its in-availability can lead to neurodegeneration.

Recent research has demonstrated that alteration in autophagic pathway can result in the formation of abnormal proteins. This is commonly observed in neurodegenerative diseases, such as Alzheimer's, Huntington's and Parkinson's diseases. In addition, many of the proteins related to Parkinson's disease, such as PINK1 and PARKIN, have an important role in the process of autophagy. Autophagy is part of the cell's self-maintenance machinery. Thus, maintaining a proper level of autophagy is important for reducing abnormal protein aggregates.

Discovery of drugs/substances that can boost autophagic activity could significantly reduce neuronal loss, preventing the progression of the disease. A clearer understanding of the regulatory processes involved in autophagic pathogenesis of PD will facilitate the identification of feasible methods for clinical application.

Alzheimer's disease

Alzheimer's disease is a progressive neurodegenerative disorder that causes brain cells and tissues to degenerate. Alzheimer's disease is the number one cause of dementia. It influences thinking, behavioral and social skills making the affected person to appear confused.

Affected individuals have a tendency to forget recent events and conversations. In later stages, patients suffering from Alzheimer's disease will develop severe memory impairment (sometimes permanent impairment) and might find it difficult to perform everyday tasks.

Treatment might temporarily improve symptoms or reduce the rate of decline. These treatments are very useful for patients suffering from Alzheimer's disease as they can help them improve the quality of their life, helping them maintain independence for some time. Modern programs and services have been created to help support patients with Alzheimer's disease and their caregivers.

Like many other neurodegenerative diseases, Alzheimer's disease is not curable at the present time. Alzheimer’s disease alters brain function and can cause in advanced stages severe complications such as loss of brain function, dehydration, malnutrition, infection and even death.

Symptoms

Memory loss is the predominant symptom of Alzheimer's disease. The first symptom of the disease is usually difficulty to remember recent events and conversations. Total or partial memory loss might result later.

At first, people with Alzheimer's disease may be aware of their shortcomings (newfound forgetfulness).

Brain alterations associated with Alzheimer's disease lead to growing trouble with memory. We all have occasional lapses in memory. It's normal to lose track of one or two things from time to time. The memory loss associated with Alzheimer's disease is different. It often persists and worsens with time, affecting a person’s ability to carry out tasks independently.

Individuals suffering from Alzheimer’s disease would routinely exhibit the following:

-Forget discussions/conversations, forget events and even names of family members (children, spouses, siblings) or even forget them totally.

-Casually misplace possessions, usually putting them in obscure places.

-Usually make poor conversations. They might find it difficult to make out sentences or reason out words. They always seem to be in a world of their own.

In relation to their thoughts and reasoning, they might exhibit the following:

-Might find it difficult to concentrate on a particular thing.

-Multitasking becomes nearly impossible. Patients usually forget important things. Alzheimer patients should not be left on their own. There should always be someone around them.

-The ability to make rational decisions and judgments declines gradually. Patients might make unusual or uncharacteristic choices such as social interactions and choice of clothing.

-Might find it difficult to perform routine tasks or activities like cooking, playing games and even grooming (dressing and bathing).

Patients might have changes in behavior or character. Patients might exhibit the following:

-Seasonal depression,

-Social withdrawal,

-Frequent mood swings,

-Becoming very suspicious (develop theories),

-Increased aggression,

-Unusual sleeping patterns, -

Wandering about or getting lost, -

Unpredictability.

Memorized skills

Memorized skills are kept for longer periods of time, even in the latter stages of the disease. Memorized skills may include studying, defense, storytelling, singing, listening to music, dancing, drawing and sculpting.

Researchers say these skills are preserved longer because they are governed by paths of the brain that only become affected when the disease worsens.

If you experience any of these symptoms, consider seeing a doctor.

Causes

There is no designated cause. However, scientists think the disease results from a combination of genetic, lifestyle and environmental factors that alter the brain's normal functioning.

A meager one percent of Alzheimer's cases is caused by genetic alterations. Individuals that display these alterations are more likely to develop the disease. Alzheimer's caused by genetic alterations usually has a quick onset (middle age occurrence).

The precise causes of Alzheimer's disease are yet to be discovered. Scientists only know that the disease results from damages (usually permanent) to the brain. This disrupts the work of brain cells (neurons) and causes a series of toxic events. Neurons are damaged, and usually lose previous connections to each other and eventually die.

The damage generally begins in the area of the brain that controls memory. However, the actual process usually starts years before the first symptoms appear. The loss of neurons is a major characteristic of the disease and it soon spreads to other parts of the brain. Towards the later stages of the disease, the brain shrinks considerably.

Like most diseases related to autophagy, scientists believe that altered proteins play a major role in its occurrence. Beta-amyloid is a product of a larger protein. When these smaller protein fragments come together, they seem to have a toxic effect on the body's neurons and contribute to cell-tocell communication disruption.

These clusters join together forming larger deposits called amyloid plaques. Proteins play a major role in the neurons' internal support and transport system. They help carry nutrients and other essential materials to the neurons. In Alzheimer's disease, proteins change shape and join together forming structures known as neurofibrillary tangles. These tangles disrupt the body's transport systems and are toxic to the cells.

Lifestyle and heart health

Recent studies have shown that heart disease and Alzheimer's disease share similar predisposing factors. These factors include:

-Lack of exercise/sedentary lifestyle,

-Smoking or continuous exposure to secondhand smoke,

-High blood pressure,

-High cholesterol,

-Poor management of type 2 diabetes.

It should be noted that many of these factors can equally reduce autophagy.

Living a healthy life can help reduce the chances of developing Alzheimer's disease. Studies have shown an association between mental engagement

and the disease. People who engaged their brains more where less likely to develop it.

Alzheimer's disease and autophagy

Alzheimer's is not a preventable disease. However, a healthy lifestyle, especially one that promotes autophagy has proven to be very helpful. Elements of autophagy such as proper exercising, healthy diets (ketosis) and adequate sleep have proven to be very beneficial to patients. Many of the factors that help prevent the disease (as recommended by doctors/medical personnel) are similar to those that stimulate autophagy.

Autophagy equally helps prevent the formation of abnormal proteins. Scientists believe that these abnormal proteins are the cause/reason neurons get damaged. Autophagy also helps to correct malformed proteins.

Furthermore, autophagy is very effective in reducing the effect of the disease in ongoing sufferers/patients (palliative).

Prion disease

This is another neurodegenerative disease. However, Prion disease is an infectious neurodegenerative disorder. Prion disease is also known as transmissible spongiform encephalopathies (TSEs). It is a zoonotic disease (can affect humans and animals). Prions are infectious agents responsible for many fatal diseases.

Prions occur in different forms. Some examples of prions that occur in humans are kuru, Creutzfeldt–Jakob disease, Gerstmann–Sträussler–Scheinker syndrome and fatal familial insomnia. In animals, the most predominant prion is the scrapie disease. It is a zoonotic disease (transmissible to humans).

Prion diseases are known for their long incubation periods and central nervous system spongiosis. Prion spongiosis is associated with neuronal loss that alters the normal brain tissue structure. The disease has a quick onset of action and is classified as chronic. In severe cases prion can cause brain damage and even death. Symptoms may include dementia, convulsions, ataxia and behavioral changes.

Prion disease and autophagy

Prion diseases are characterized by spongiform degeneration. They induce the accumulation of misfolded and aggregated PrP (altered proteins) in the central nervous system. The symptoms are usually fatal (list of symptoms above) and neurodegeneration caused by this disease is severe. Recent studies have shown that autophagy vacuoles in neurons were frequently detected in neurodegenerative prion diseases.

Scientists consider that autophagy plays an important role in the elimination of pathological PrP (altered proteins) accumulated within neurons. Likewise, autophagy dysfunction in affected body neurons may result in the formation of spongiform changes.

Amyotrophic Lateral Sclerosis (ALS)

Amyotrophic Lateral Sclerosis (ALS) is a neurodegenerative disorder characterized by a gradual loss of motor neurons (both upper and lower motor neurons) in the central nervous system (C.N.S). The disorder is usually very severe and occurs mostly in elderly patients.

Statistically, Amyotrophic Lateral Sclerosis (ALS) is the most common motor neuron disorder in the world. It has an incidence rate of 2.7 per 100,000 and an age-of-onset varying between 50–65 years.

Symptoms include spasticity, quadriplegia and muscle atrophy. Patients usually die within 3-5 years (following onset of the disease). Normally, respiratory failure is the last complication to occur before death.

Available drugs include Riluzole, which prolongs survival by 2–3 months in some patients, and Radicava which helps to prevent decline in physical function. Like most neurodegenerative diseases, Amyotrophic Lateral Sclerosis has no cure.

The disease has two forms. These are the familial ALS (fALS) and sporadic ALS (sALS). sALS is the predominant form, comprising 90%–95% of the cases. sALS does not have any known genetic links. However, fALS affects 5%–10% of the cases (it has hereditary links).

Like many of its counterparts (neurodegenerative disorders), sclerosis exhibits the usual mis-localization of body proteins and the presence of cytoplasmic aggregates in motor neurons. This again points to an alteration in the body's protein metabolism.

Amyotrophic Lateral Sclerosis (ALS) and autophagy

An important pathological feature of ALS is the accumulation of insoluble protein aggregates in degenerating motor neurons and surrounding cells in the central nervous system.

These protein aggregates are typically formed by misfolded proteins that have been altered. The formation of misfolded protein aggregates is not totally pathological. It occurs naturally in the body (the body's cells continuously employ control mechanisms to either lyse the altered proteins to avoid aggregation or clear aggregates that have already formed).

Scientists believe that the persistence of these protein aggregates in diseased neurons suggests a disruption in autophagy. Autophagy is normally responsible for degrading/lysing altered proteins in the body. When autophagy is not functioning properly, this protein aggregate is causing harm to the body's motor neurons. Amyotrophic Lateral Sclerosis (ALS) disease usually kicks off from here.

In both forms of Amyotrophic Lateral Sclerosis (familial ALS (fALS) and sporadic ALS (sALS)), immunofluorescence studies of post-mortem (dead) brain and spinal cord tissues have shown the presence of these proteins within aggregates.

Scientist believe that autophagy is the leading light (only chance of breakthrough) in respect to developing a lasting cure to the disease.

CHAPTER FIVE

How autophagy helps you build a stronger immune system

To effectively understand the numerous ways autophagy benefits the body, a clear understanding of the human immune system is required. The body cannot do without the human immune system. Without an immune system, the body would fall into the grasp of bacteria, viruses, parasites, and more. It is the human immune system that keeps us healthy and safe from various contaminants.

This immune system consists of a vast network of cells, tissues and organs. Its components (cells, tissues and organs) are constantly searching for pathogens. Once a pathogen is located, the body mounts an organized response against it.

The human immune system is spread around the body and is made up of different proteins, cells, tissues and organs. It can distinguish self from nonself (self refers to substances/particles/molecules that are homogenous/manufactured by the body, while non-self refers to those substances/particles/molecules that are foreign to the body). The latter are also called immunogenic substances.

When the human immune system encounters a pathogen (e.g. a virus or fungi), it mounts a response. This response is known as an immunogenic response. Below are a few important immune components.

White blood cells: also called leukocytes, white bloods cells patrol the body's blood vessels as well as the lymphatic system. Much like policemen, they patrol the nooks and crannies of the body, searching for pathogens. *(Autophagy boosts their effectiveness and enhances their actions).*

They can also trigger alarm bells. Once they encounter a pathogen, they send numerous messages/signals to other body cells. The storage of white blood cells is done in lymphoid organs. Examples of lymphoid organs are:

-*Thymus:* a gland located in the middle of the lungs and slightly beneath the neck.

-*Spleen:* the organ responsible for blood filtration, found in the abdomen.

-*Bone marrow:* Very important part of the body's hematopoietic system (blood producing system). The bone marrow produces both of the blood cells.

-*Lymph nodes:* small glands found in strategic places all throughout the human body. Lymph nodes around the body are linked together through the lymphatic vessels.

There are two main types of white blood cells (leukocytes). The first type is:

Phagocytes : They are also called antigen presenting cells (antigen presenting cells are cells that present antigens to the body for destruction). They surround and break down pathogens. There are several types, including:

- *Neutrophils:* these are the most abundant type of phagocyte. They attack bacteria and other pathogens.
- *Monocytes:* they are the largest phagocytes and are very effective antigen presenting cells.
- *Macrophages:* are also antigen presenting cells. They also remove dead and dying cells.
- *Mast cells:* they are multipurpose cells. They help to heal wounds and defend against pathogens.

The second type of white blood cells is the ***lymphocytes***.

They are also called memory cells. This is because they memorize previous history or attacks by pathogens.

Lymphocytes begin a cycle in the bone marrow. Those that stay in the bone marrow grow to become B cells, and those that leave the bone marrow (head to the thymus) are called the T cells. T lymphocytes and B lymphocytes have different functions:

B lymphocytes: produce antibodies and help alert the T lymphocytes.

T lymphocytes: are known as the action lymphocytes. They destroy compromised cells in the body. They equally help to alert other lymphocytes.

What is an immune response?

B lymphocytes secrete antibodies that attack and neutralize antigens. To successfully do this, the human immune system needs to be able to differentiate self-antigens from non-self-antigens. The body starts this process very early. It encodes all its internal cells (memorizes their details).

An antigen is any substance that can initiate/spark an immune response. Examples of antigens are bacteria, fungi, virus and toxins. Sometimes altered cells and old cells can become antigens too. All components of the human immune system work together to achieve immunity (combined effort/teamwork).

The importance of B lymphocytes

B lymphocytes are very important in the body's defense against antigens. Once B lymphocytes detect an antigen, they secrete antibodies. Antibodies are special proteins produced by the body. They are specific in action (specific antibodies lock up or attack specific antigens).

For example, a specific antibody is produced by the B lymphocytes in response to mycobacterium tuberculosis. This antibody would be different from that produced against pneumonia.

Antibodies are members of a big group of chemicals known as immunoglobulins. Immunoglobulins play an important role in the body's defense against antigens. Examples of immunoglobulins are:

- Immunoglobulin G (IgG): marks microbes for easy recognition by body cells,
- IgM: attacks bacteria (major function),
- IgA: found in body fluids, such as tears as well as saliva, where it protects pathogens from entering the human body,
- IgE: guides the body from parasites. It is equally implicated in most allergies,
- IgD: initiates most body immune responses.

Antibodies do not kill or destroy antigens. Instead they lock antigens, and flag them off for destruction (destruction by phagocytes).

The importance of T lymphocytes

These are often regarded as the most important cells of the human immune system. They are divided into two: the normal T cells and the killer T cells.

Normal T cells : they direct the response given by the immune system. They interact with members of other cells (call them to the site of attack), stimulate B lymphocytes (to secret more antibodies) and draw a number of T-cells when necessary.

Killer T cells (also known as cytotoxic T lymphocytes): they are also known as fighter T-cells. They attack pathogens, especially viruses. They are the most competent cells in the body for this task. They recognize small concentrations of the virus on the surface of infected body cells. After recognition, they get rid of cells already infected.

Immunodeficiency

This is keenly discussed in modern medicine. Immunodeficiency arises when a component or components of the human immune system do not function. Immunodeficiency can result from a number of situations. These include obesity, age, malnutrition and alcoholism. AIDS is an example of an acquired immunodeficiency.

In some cases (very rare), immunodeficiency can be inherited (e.g. in chronic granulomatous disease where phagocytic function is impaired).

Autoimmunity

Autoimmune reactions are rare. In autoimmune conditions, the human immune system targets healthy body cells rather than immunogen/pathogens or faulty cells. In this condition (autoimmune disorder) they cannot distinguish self from non-self.

Autoimmune diseases include type 1 diabetes, celiac disease, Graves' disease and rheumatoid disease.

With this basic knowledge of the human immune system, the benefits of autophagy to the human immune system will be better understood. Recent experiments/research (using lab rats -MOUAU):

Resistance to disease (rats exposed to an autophagic lifestyle - Rats A)	Normal rats (not exposed to autophagy - Rats B)
Very high	Average
Immune cells - very active	Average

Rats A - Susceptibility to experimental pathogen (common flu)	Rats B - Susceptibility to experimental pathogen	Recovery rate of infected (Rats A)	Recovery rate of infected (Rats B)
30%	60%	High	Average
		Very fast	Much slower

This table creates a clearer picture of these benefits, although further details are given below.

Boosting the human immune system through autophagy

One of the major means of achieving autophagy (fasting) has proven to be one of the most effective ways of boosting immunity.

Recent research has shown that fasting for 72 hours induces immune system regeneration.

Fasting for 72 hours (3 days) can regenerate the entire immune system and reverse the damage done to the human immune system by chemotherapy.

Previously, fasting was regarded as bad or unhealthy. However, modern research results suggest that starving the body stimulates stem cells to produce new white blood cells, which defend the body in times of infection.

Recent research has shown that prolonged fasting can have a remarkable effect in promoting stem cell-based regeneration of the hematopoietic system. When the body is starved, it tries to save energy, and one of the things it can do to save energy is to recycle a lot of the immune cells that are damaged or redundant.

The findings from this research are revolutionary. With a renewed/boosted immune system, the chances of a long and healthy life are increased.

In fact, yogis and sages have done this in past times. Western medicine is only embracing it now.

How fasting stimulates the human immune system

Fasting is one of the pillars of autophagy. Prolonged fasting forces the body to utilize its stores of glucose, fat and ketones. It also breaks down a significant portion of lymphocytes/white blood cells (broken down for new cells to be generated).

In each fasting cycle there is a depletion of lymphocytes. This causes changes that stimulate stem cell-based regeneration of new immune system cells.

After fasting there is a reduction in the production of the enzyme PKA, a body hormone known to cause an increased risk of cancer and tumor growth. In addition, the human immune system of the subject (research done on animals) appeared to be boosted.

Prolonged fasting can reduce the harmful effects of chemotherapy

Prolonged fasting helps to protect the body from toxicity. This is an amazing development, especially for cancer patients who adopt chemotherapy as their treatment choice.

Chemotherapy remains one of the best ways to treat cancer. However, it causes significant collateral damage to the human immune system. The results obtained from this study suggest that fasting can reduce some of the harmful effects of chemotherapy.

The amazing benefits of fasting are not limited to the human immune system. Scientists believe these effects are applicable to many different conditions, systems and organs in the body.

Additional benefits of prolonged fasting

Scientists are beginning to discover more benefits of fasting. Below are some of these amazing benefits.

You will likely experience weight loss. First, you will lose weight because you lose water and stored products like glycogen. This is why increasing water consumption during prolonged fasting is important. In any case, depleting your glycogen levels will induce an artificial state of ketosis, turning the body into a fat burning machine.

Your body will "start to eat itself". This predictably leads to autophagy. Autophagy removes waste from the body and repairs any oxidative stress.

You brain activity increases with prolonged fasting. This makes sense when you think about it. When we were hunters and gatherers and we hadn't eaten for a few days, we needed to come up with new ideas in order to find more food: our ability to think critically has improved in these situations. Some research shows that ketosis benefits the brain, resulting in more brain-derived neurotrophic factor or BDNF.

Is prolonged fasting the same as intermittent fasting?

Intermittent fasting means submitting your body to a schedule of prolonged fasting (regulating your food intake over a period of time).

An individual may fast for 16 hours per day, only consuming food within an

8-hour window (eating between 11 am and 7 pm, fasting between 7 pm and 11 am the next day). Doing this repeatedly, or 5 days per week, means you are adopting an intermittent fasting schedule.

Prolonged fasting usually refers to fasting for a longer period. This is usually for about 2 days or more.

Autophagy and HIV

Recent research has shown that autophagy plays a role in preventing the replication and progression of the HIV virus. Autophagy was found to protect the small proportion of HIV-1 infected individuals who remain clinically stable for years in the absence of antiretroviral therapy. It boosts immunity (generates a constant supply of proteins to the immune cells). This gives them the needed boost and reinforcement they require to fight the disease.

Autophagy can be likened to an arms dealer (in the body) that supplies arms free of charge (to fight off HIV).

What is HIV

Before we discuss the amazing benefits of autophagy in respect to HIV, we will have a short rundown of the disease.

HIV is a virus that destroys (technically) the human immune system. The human immune system helps the body in its defense (from different pathogens - viruses, bacteria and opportunistic infections). Untreated, it infects and kills CD4 cells, which are a type of immune cell called T cells. Over time, HIV kills more CD4 cells. This makes the body prone to opportunistic infections (CD4 cells are very important defense cells).

As always, we shall discuss its mode of transmission, symptoms, diagnosis and treatment. Knowing the above is becoming more and more important nowadays.

HIV is transmitted through bodily fluids that include:

- blood,
- semen,
- vaginal and rectal fluids,
- breastmilk.

HIV can be transmitted or spread through different means. These include:

- through vaginal or anal sex (this is the most common route of transmission, especially among men who have sex with men),
- by sharing needles, syringes, and other items for injection drug use,
- by sharing tattoo equipment without sterilizing it between uses,
- during pregnancy, labor, or delivery from a woman to her baby,
- during breastfeeding,
- through "pre-mastication," or chewing a baby's food before feeding it to them,
- through exposure to the blood of a person living with HIV, such as through a needle stick.

The virus can also be transmitted through a blood transfusion or organ and tissue transplant. However, rigorous testing for the virus among blood, organ and tissue donors ensures that this is very rare in the United States.

It's theoretically possible to get infected through exposure to the blood of someone living with HIV, such as through a needle stick, but it is a rare occurrence for HIV to spread through:

- oral sex (only if there are bleeding gums or open sores in the person's mouth),
- being bitten by a person with HIV (only if the saliva is bloody or there are open sores in the person's mouth),
- contact between broken skin, wounds, or mucous membranes and the blood of someone living with HIV.

HIV is a lifelong condition and currently no cure is available, although many scientists are working hard to find one. However, with medical treatment (antiretroviral therapy) and a *healthy lifestyle (autophagy-based lifestyle),* it is possible to manage HIV and live forward with the virus.

HIV lowers the body's CD4 cell count, weakening the human immune system. A normal adult's CD4 count is 500 to 1,500 per cubic millimeter. An individual with a count below 200 is considered to have AIDS. **Research has shown that, when combined with an effective treatment, autophagy can help maintain the CD4 count in infected individuals.**

It's important to note that if an infected person is being treated and has a persistently undetectable viral load, it is virtually impossible to transmit the virus to another person.

Early symptoms of HIV can include:

- Night fever
- Body chills
- Swollen lymph nodes
- Body aches and pains
- Skin rash
- Sore throat
- Headache
- Nausea
- Running stomach

Prevention

The most common way of transmission (HIV) is through anal or vaginal sex without a condom. This risk can't be completely eliminated unless sex is avoided altogether. However, the risk can be lowered considerably by taking a few precautions. These precautions include:

- *Regular testing/checkups:* Knowing your status and that of those around you is very important.

Get tested for other sexually transmitted infections (STIs). If you test positive for one, you should get it treated immediately, because having an STI increases the risk of infection (contracting HIV).

- *Use condoms:* If you must have sex, especially with a partner you do not trust, you should learn the correct way to use condoms and use them every time you have sex, whether it's vaginal or anal intercourse. It's important to note that pre-seminal fluids (which come out before male ejaculation) can contain HIV.

- *Have only one partner:* This reduces the chances of getting infected.

Promiscuity increases the chances.

Take your medications as directed if you have been infected. This lowers the risk of transmitting the virus or developing complications.

If you are sexually active, you should always ensure that you have condoms around.

Autophagy and HIV

Autophagy diets help reduce the effects of HIV on the body. It is not only limited to HIV (it applies to other diseases too). It also promotes healthy aging and reduces risk of heart disease, diabetes and cancer.

HIV is a chronic inflammatory condition, further stressing the already weakening immune system that accompanies aging. Dietary protein, trace minerals and antioxidant nutrients help to slow the rate of aging and can help prevent frailty.

Immune cell functions are sensitive to nutrition deficits. HIV infection alters gut microflora, impeding all nutrient absorption.

Nutrition is about providing materials needed by the body in its day to day operations. The balance between fats, proteins, fruits and carbs differs slightly from the normal autophagy diet.

An autophagy-based diet for someone with HIV should contain more fish and seafood and less meat than other diets. There should be liberal amounts of fruit and vegetables, including many wild greens in the diet. Whole grains such as cereals and sourdough bread are recommended. HIV patients should avoid pasta. Legumes, rich in magnesium, should be eaten almost daily. Fats should come from nuts, olives and olive oil. Dairy should be consumed more in the form of cheese than milk. Goat and sheep milk cheeses are recommended. Chemically, the diet should contain more selenium and glutathione, plus a healthier balance of omega-6 to omega-3 fats. The diet should equally be rich in antioxidants like vitamins C and E, plus resveratrol from red grapes/wine, and the anti-inflammatory oleuropein (obtained from olive oil).

Tips for Assembling a Healthy Autophagy Diet in HIV

-Choose healthy protein foods and eat them three times a day. *Unlike in the normal autophagy diet, HIV patients need more protein.*

The American Heart Association recommends two 4-ounce servings per week of oily fish. Statistically, very few people consume fish in a week, so a daily fish oil pill supplement should be considered. Up to 6 grams a day of fish oils have reduced triglyceride levels by almost 40% in an HIV population.

Research has shown that whey protein powder is a useful and cheap additive to a meal. It is often added to breakfast cereal or protein-fruit smoothies. Trials of whey protein in HIV populations' diets have shown that it can boost the human immune system and reverse glutathione (antioxidant enzyme) deficiency. Whey can also improve bone strength (prevent joint pain or other non-related conditions). Consumed dairy products should be fat-free or low-fat.

-Add lots of vegetables to your diet for both lunch and dinner. Three cups a day should be the minimum amount to eat. This is needed in order to obtain Cretan-diet levels of minerals and phytochemicals. HIV-infected people consuming a dietary pattern that included a higher intake of vegetables, fruits and low-fat dairy foods usually develop a stronger and more effective immune system.

-Try eating fruit three times a day to increase glutathione and glutathione peroxidase levels. Eating fruit, including the traditional "apple-a-day," provides the body with water-soluble fiber (pectin). This aids the growth of beneficial gut flora, which lowers cholesterol levels, C-reactive protein levels and body percent fat.

-Nuts and seeds contain important oils that form cell membranes. You should try to eat a handful of nuts and one of seeds every day. **These oils**

help improve autophagy in the body (they help to rebuild the body and help boost the human immune system).

-Starches (carbohydrates) are the remaining part of fuel and food needs. Legumes, technically a protein-rich starch, are an important component of the HIV autophagy diet (however, the quantity of carbs should be reduced), providing fiber, plant protein and magnesium. Higher magnesium consumption is inversely related to cardiac and cancer mortality. More than half of the grains consumed should be whole grains. Whole grains are generally recommended as a carbohydrate source.

In addition to creating a diet that focuses on variety, nutrient density, and amounts, the calories from added sugars and saturated fats, along with sodium should be limited/reduced drastically.

Other healthy products to achieve autophagy (in HIV patients)

- *Coconut oil:* is a reliable autophagy inducer. Coconut oil is growing in popularity around the world. This is because of its endless benefits. Coconut oil has been found to be beneficial by doctors, weight loss experts, nutritionists and many other professionals. The benefits of coconut oil are so many that only a few can be discussed.

One of the major uses of coconut oil in modern times is in weight loss. Unlike many other oils or fats, coconut oil is made up of medium chain fatty acids. Medium chain fatty acids, as opposed to long chain fatty acids, are metabolized in the liver, before being broken down to ketone bodies. This simply implies that coconut oil supplies the body with a large amount of energy, thus restricting the urge and need to eat subsequently. This helps prevent the consumption of in-between meals that cause weight gain (excess weight gain for an HIV patient is not healthy).

Still on weight loss, coconut oil is also thermogenic. Thus, it stimulates the burning of fat in the body. Although coconut oil is not very aggressive in causing weight loss, it is very helpful when taken over a period of time and is very helpful in removing belly fat. Other benefits of coconut oil include improving cardiogenic function and overall health of the heart, treatment and palliative remedy for Alzheimer's disease, keeping the skin and hair healthy and radiant, maintaining dental health, improving the body's immunity, reducing inflammation thanks to its anti-inflammatory properties and improving gut health and digestion.

-*Good wine: Yes! Who says HIV patients can't have some fun?* From the olden times and until now, wines have remained very popular. They are classy and when prepared well give a quality luxurious taste. Wines are not just luxurious drinks (as most of us see them). They possess numerous health benefits. Some of these benefits include antioxidative properties which prevent cancer. Wine equally promotes bone health, especially in elderly people, reduces the risk of stroke, has positive cardiogenic effect, reduces body cholesterol levels and helps to prevent diabetes. It is therefore safe to say that, when consumed adequately or in controlled quantities, wine can benefit the body greatly. *To cap it up, wine can equally induce autophagy (although mildly).*

Autophagy diets for the elderly (elderly people with HIV)

Reduced antioxidant activity coupled with mitochondrial damage underlie the faster rates of deterioration occurring in this population.

Common health conditions encountered in the elderly population include osteoporosis, vascular disease risk, sarcopenia, loss of cognitive function, fatigue/frailty and immune deficiency.

Subtle nutrient deficiencies can cause all of these problems. Using comprehensive nutrition therapy to treat HIV offers the opportunity to avoid increased pharmacologic burden in a population where side effects are pronounced.

The diet should contain fish, at least twice a week.

Vitamin supplements and natural calcium sources are usually not enough to strengthen weakening bones. In recent experiments, an algae-derived calcium was used, with strontium, boron, magnesium supplements, as well as vitamins D and K2 and the result was that osteoporosis was reversed in only 6-12 months in older populations (older HIV patients).

Safety measures can reduce falls at home and increased fitness levels can lower fracture rates. Equally, eating soft bones (biscuit bones) is very helpful, as it improves muscle action and helps improve body energy levels.

Consume lots of fruits and vegetables: An autophagy diet for elderly HIV patients should contain lots of vegetables and fruits. This would supply them with the necessary nutrients and vitamins needed to ward off infection.

Patients need to be reminded of the importance of positive lifestyle factors such as eating healthy, proper nutrition, and fitness in maintaining their health and improve the quality of their life while aging with HIV.

Food and *fitness education* can reduce complications in aged HIV population by 75% over two decades.

Multivitamin supplements boost the human immune system generally and are highly recommended for elderly HIV patients.

Autophagy based exercise

Exercise cannot control or fight HIV disease, but it is palliative and fights against many of the side effects of HIV disease or HIV medications. It can help you live a healthy life despite being infected with HIV.

What are the advantages of exercise ?

Regular/daily exercise has the same advantages for people with HIV disease as it does for most people. Exercise can:

- Improve muscle condition
- Improve heart and lung performance
- Increase your energy level so you feel less tired
- Reduce stress
- Enhance the body's well-being
- Increase bone strength
- Reduce cholesterol levels
- Increase good (HDL) cholesterol
- Reduce body fat
- Improve appetite
- Improve sleep

Reduce blood sugar levels

Exercise guidelines for people with HIV

A moderate exercise program will improve your body fitness and minimize health risks. At first, go slow and schedule exercise into your daily routines.

For starters, work up a schedule of at least 20 minutes, three times per week to the best of your abilities. This can lead to significant improvements in your fitness level and make you healthier. As your strength, stamina and energy increase, try to aim at 45 minutes to an hour, three to four times a week.

People with HIV can improve their body fitness levels through training like those who do not have HIV. However, people with HIV may find it difficult to continue because of fatigue.

Vary your routine so that you do not get bored. Find new ways to keep yourself stimulated to maintain your exercise program. Finding an exercise mate might help keep you motivated.

As your stamina might be reduced (following infection), it is very important that you work your way gradually. As little as 10 minutes is good enough until you build up to an hour. *Exercise induces autophagy and it brings all these benefits to HIV sufferers.*

Exercise with weights

Lifting weights is the most effective form of exercise (in respect to autophagy). Weight training (resistance exercise) is one of the best ways to increase lean body mass and bone density that may be lost through HIV disease. Working out three times a week for an hour should be enough if done properly. Doing weight training followed by 30 minutes of cardiovascular exercise may be the most effective way to improve body composition and keep your blood lipids and sugar down. Cardiovascular exercise means increasing oxygen supply to the body and heart rate while moving large muscle groups continuously for at least 30 minutes. Brisk walking, jogging, dancing, bicycling or swimming are all examples of cardiovascular exercise. Be creative about ways not to remain sedentary. The quality of your life depends on this!

An autophagy-based exercise program can improve lean body mass, reduce fat, stress, weakness and depression, improve strength, stamina and cardiovascular fitness. It can also boost the human immune system (make it perform better).

Autophagy and Tuberculosis

What is Tuberculosis?

Tuberculosis, also known as TB, is a very contagious infection, which most often affects the human lungs, and can be quickly spread to other parts of one's body, including the brain, without proper treatment. It is caused by mycobacterium tuberculosis.

In the 20's, tuberculosis was a leading cause of death worldwide. Today, a lot of prevalent TB cases are treated with antibiotics. However, recovery (cure) takes a longer amount of time, the treatment involving taking drugs for a period of six to twelve months.

In What Ways Can Tuberculosis Affect Your Body?

Getting infected doesn't automatically make you ill. The disease comes in two different forms:

-*Latent TB:* In this case, the virus is prevalent in your body, but it is in a constant battle with your immune system, which tries to prevent it from getting to other parts of your body. There would be no symptoms and the carrier would not be considered contagious. However, the disease still lives in the carrier's body and someday it might become active. If the carrier poses a high risk for the disease to become active, for instance people with HIV, the doctor would have you placed on antibiotics to reduce the chances of your TB becoming active. **People with a strong immune system and those who live a healthy lifestyle (autophagy lifestyle) usually fall in this category. Most times they are able to withstand the infection. The infection usually wears off with time.**

-*Active TB disease:* The body is not able to control the disease. Those with active TB usually fall ill. More than 2/3 of adult cases of active TB result from the reactivation of a latent TB infection.

Symptoms of Tuberculosis

There aren't any symptoms for latent TB. You would need to get a skin or blood test to know if you're infected.

Signs of an active TB disease include:

- Persistent cough
- Chest pain
- Coughing up blood
- Weakness
- Night sweats
- Chills
- Fever
- Loss of appetite
- Weight loss

If you experience any of these symptoms, see your doctor to get tested.

Mode of transmission

The disease is airborne, just like catching a cold or getting hit by flu. Anything that involves fluid from any already infected person, like a quick cough, a sneeze, loud talks and laughter or any other thing that can cause saliva to leave the mouth, is one way the disease can be spread. This is due to the fact that saliva contains traces of the bacteria. Once you are unlucky enough to take in the bacteria (through any of the above), you can get infected.

Tuberculosis is considered very contagious but getting infected is not that easy. To get infected, you would be required to be around someone who is already infected for quite some time. This person still has to have a high level of bacilli load in their lungs. The need for proximity is one major reason it is quickly passed among people who spend time with each other.

Tuberculosis bacteria rarely survives on plane surfaces. Therefore, one cannot become a carrier simply by exchanging body contact or by partaking the food and drinks of someone who is already infected.

Risk factors

You can only get TB through contact with an infected person. Here are some factors that could increase your risk:

- A friend, co-worker or family member is infected.
- You live or have traveled to a TB endemic region like Russia, Africa, Eastern Europe, Asia, Latin America and the Caribbean.
- You are part of a group where TB is easily transmitted, or you work or live with someone who is. Members of this exposed group include homeless people, HIV patients and IV drug users. • You work or live in a hospital.

The role of an autophagic diet in recovery from tuberculosis

While the treatment of active tuberculosis is long term – up to a year of daily antibiotics – you can aid your recovery and help your body fight off the disease by making sure it gets an adequate nutrition. Your body needs healthy nutrients now more than ever.

People who are malnourished or underweight are more likely to get infected with tuberculosis and are also more susceptible to reinfection or relapse of TB after treatment. Malnutrition leads to decreased immunity, and your body needs to be as strong as possible to defend itself against tuberculosis bacteria.

Poor nutrition can actually encourage the persistence of tuberculosis, and this can lead to malnutrition. Therefore, to help your body fight TB, you have to feed it correctly.

To arm your body with the nutrients it needs to defeat tuberculosis and regain your strength and stamina, you need to eat a diet containing a variety of healthy foods (autophagy diet), such as:

- Vegetables, for their high iron and B-vitamin content.
-

Reasonable quantity of carbohydrates, like whole wheat pastas, breads and cereals (in reduced quantity). In all autophagy diets carbohydrates are reduced.

- Colored vegetables such as carrots, peppers and squash. Fruits like tomatoes, blueberries and cherries. Colored vegetables are rich in antioxidants.
- Unsaturated fats like vegetable or olive oil instead of coconut oil or butter. Unsaturated fat has tremendous benefits (especially to tuberculosis patients). Unsaturated fats are very useful, especially when they consign achieving autophagy.

Talk to your doctor about whether or not you have any nutrient deficiencies and if taking in daily multivitamins with minerals is necessary. A recent review of the limited studies done on supplements in patients with TB showed that high-calorie energy supplements helped underweight patients gain body weight, and that zinc, when taken with other micronutrients or with vitamin A, may offer nutritional help.

Avoid:

Generally, what is unhealthy remains unhealthy. Similarly, what is healthy remains healthy. Thus, a risk factor for tuberculosis can equally apply to several other diseases. Steps to be taken in order to limit these risks include:

- Avoiding smoking or tobacco.
- Avoiding alcohol. This can add to the risk of liver damage from some of the drugs used to treat your TB.
- Reducing consumption of coffee and other caffeinated drinks.
- Limiting refined carbohydrates like sugar, white breads and white rice (they limit autophagy - cellular regeneration).
- Avoid high-fat, high-cholesterol red meat and instead consume leaner protein sources like poultry, beans, tofu and fish.

Strive to give your body the nutrition it needs to maintain a healthy weight and build up body strength to destroy the tuberculosis bacteria and reduce your risk of a relapse. Eating a nutritious/healthy diet and staying away from unhealthy habits will help you feel better, faster.

Exercise

By now, you should know that exercise is one of the ways to achieve autophagy. People who are suffering from tuberculosis may have difficulty in performing physical exercise and being inactive during the lengthy treatment can make you feel weak. However, physical activity can speed recovery and help you manage your weight.

Recent research has shown that exercise can help the body fight the TB infection and not only speed your recovery but also improve your mood. If you have inactive TB, you can continue your normal exercise routines. You need a doctor's approval to perform or carry out any physical training if you have active TB. Moderate walking is a good way to start, especially if you are not used to exercise.

Start with short sessions, such as walking for 20 minutes. With time and frequency, your stamina will increase. You should walk as often as possible. As you build your stamina, you can increase your walking time gradually. Once active TB is no longer transmittable, if you feel well enough and your doctor approves, you should be able to return to your normal workout routines.

CHAPTER SIX

Autophagy and Cancer

Cancer causes cells to divide without control. This can cause tumors, damage to the body's immune system and other complications.

Cancer is a vast term. It describes the disease that results when cellular alterations induce the uncontrolled growth and division of cells.

Some types of cancer cause rapid cell multiplication, while others cause the body cells to grow and divide at a slower rate.

Certain forms of cancer can cause tumors while others, such as leukemia, do not.

The body's cells are specific in action. They have fixed lifespans. Cell death is a natural and beneficial phenomenon called apoptosis (cells die and are then replaced – autophagy).

A cell receives an order (to die) so that the body can replace it with a newer cell that functions better. Cancerous cells do not follow this order (are out of control).

As a result, they build up in the body, using oxygen and nutrients that would usually nourish other body cells. Cancerous cells can cause tumors, impair the human immune system and induce changes that prevent the body from functioning normally.

Cancerous cells may appear in one area, then spread via the lymph nodes to another part of the body.

Causes

Certain conditions or factors increase a person's chances of developing cancer. They include:

- Smoking
- Heavy alcohol consumption
- Obesity
- Sedentary lifestyle
- Malnutrition

Other causes of cancer are not preventable. Currently, the most important risk factor is age.

Genetic factors can equally add to the chances of developing cancer.

A person's genetic code controls the division of cells. Alterations in these genes can lead to faulty instructions, and cancer can result.

Genes also influence the body's protein production. Proteins carry most of the instructions for cellular growth and division.

Some genes alter proteins that would usually repair damaged cells. This can lead to cancer. If a person has a relative with these genes, the chances of that person developing cancer are higher.

Some genetic alterations occur after birth, and factors such as smoking and sun exposure can increase the risk.

Other alterations that can result in cancer take place in the chemical signals that determine how the body deploys or "expresses" specific genes.

Finally, a person can inherit predisposition for a type of cancer. Medically, this is called hereditary cancer syndrome. Inherited genetic mutations contribute to the development of about 5–10 percent of cancer cases.

Types

- Bladder
- Colon and rectal
- Endometrial

- Kidney
- Leukemia
- Liver
- Melanoma
- Non-Hodgkin's lymphoma
- Pancreatic
- Thyroid

Other forms are less common. According to the National Cancer Institute, there are over a hundred types of cancer.

Effect of autophagy on cancer (fasting)

The component of autophagy that affects cancer the most is fasting. Fasting may help with cancer treatment. There is growing proof supporting the role of fasting in both cancer treatment and prevention.

Recent research has shown that fasting helps fight cancer by lowering insulin resistance and levels of inflammation. Fasting may also reverse the effects of chronic body conditions such as obesity and type 2 diabetes, which are both risk factors for cancer.

Also, researchers believe that fasting makes cancer cells more responsive to treatment (especially chemotherapy) while protecting other cells. Fasting may also boost the human immune system to help fight or prevent its spread.

Improving insulin sensitivity

Fasting may help improve the effectiveness of chemotherapy.

Insulin is a hormone that allows cells to extract glucose from the blood and generate energy.

When food is consumed in excess, the cells in the body become less sensitive to insulin. This insulin resistance means that the cells respond to insulin signals slowly and sometimes they don't respond at all. This causes increased levels of glucose in the blood and higher fat storage.

When the food supply is scarce, the human body tries to conserve energy.

It achieves this by making cell membranes more sensitive to insulin. Cells can metabolize insulin more efficiently, removing glucose from the blood.

Better insulin sensitivity makes it difficult for cancer cells to grow or develop.

Reversing the chronic conditions

Recent research has also shown that conditions such as obesity and type 2 diabetes are risk factors for cancer. Both are linked to a higher risk of cancer and lower survival rate.

Modern research has also illustrated the effect of short-term fasting on type 2 diabetes. The participants in the study fasted for 24 hours two to three times per week.

After 4 months of fasting, the participants had a 20 percent reduction in weight and a 12 percent reduction in waist size.

Also, the participants no longer required insulin treatment after 2 months of this fasting pattern.

Improving quality of life during chemotherapy

Fasting may help reduce chemotherapy related complications.

Recent studies show that fasting improves people's response to chemotherapy because it does the following:

- promotes regeneration of all the body cells, protects blood from
- some of the harmful effects of chemotherapy, lessens the impact of
- side effects, such as fatigue, nausea, headaches and cramps.

A 2018 study showed that fasting can improve the quality of life in people undergoing chemotherapy for breast or ovarian cancer. The study was based on a 60-hour fasting period (about 36 hours before the start of chemotherapy).

The results show that those who fasted during chemotherapy reported higher tolerance to chemotherapy, fewer chemotherapy related complications and higher energy levels when compared with those who did not fast.

Boosting the human immune system to fight cancer

Fasting produces cancer-fighting effects in stem cells. Stem cells are very important in the body for their regenerative abilities.

Fasting for 2–4 days protects stem cells from some of the negative effects of chemotherapy on the human immune system.

Fasting also causes stem cells in the human immune system to regenerate.

This study shows that fasting not only limits damage to cells, it also replenishes the body.

White blood cells help the body fight infection and destroy cells that may cause disease. When white blood cell levels usually drop during chemotherapy, it affects the human immune system negatively, and the body might not be able to prevent infections.

The number of white blood cells in the blood decreases during fasting. However, when the fasting cycle concludes and the body receives food, white blood cell levels increase significantly. They almost double in number.

Cancer causes cells to divide without control. It also prevents them from dying naturally, following their normal cycle.

Genetic factors and lifestyle choices, such as smoking, can contribute to the development of cancer. Several components affect the ways the DNA communicates with cells and directs their division and death.

Treatments are constantly improving. Examples of current treatments include chemotherapy, radiation therapy and surgery. Some people benefit from more modern treatments, such as stem cell transplantation and precision medicine. However, most of these treatments are harsh and largely ineffective. Fasting (one of the pillars of autophagy) has yielded amazing results in cancer patients. Researchers believe that autophagy is the long-term solution to cancer.

Short and prolonged fasting periods have yielded amazing results in cancer treatment and prevention.

Stay young forever through autophagy

Aging is the process of becoming older. The term refers to human beings, most animals and fungi, whereas for example bacteria, perennial plants and some simple animals are technically biologically immortal. In a different light, aging can refer to single cells within an organism which have stopped dividing (cellular senescence) or to the population of a species (population aging).

In animals, aging can be described as the accumulation of changes over a particular period of time. These could be physical, psychological or social changes. For example, body movement or responsiveness may slow with age, while knowledge of world events and wisdom may increase. Aging is one of the most important risk factors in human diseases: of the roughly 150,000 people who die each day across the world, about two-thirds die from age-related causes.

Aging is a complex process characterized by the progressive failure of maintenance and repair pathways critical for cellular preservation, which results in a gradual accumulation of unwanted macromolecules and organelles. The accumulation of such oxidized, misfolded, cross-linked or aggregated molecules has negative effects on cellular homeostasis and on tissue and organ integrity. The defective molecules can alter homeostasis directly by interfering with the activity of functional molecules and organelles, which can cause further dysfunction. This progressive decline in cellular homeostasis leads to aging, disease and ultimately, to death. Although our understanding of the biology of aging has increased in recent times, the molecular events underlying this process have only recently begun to be explored. Interestingly, research in the last couple of decades focused on deciphering the molecular underpinnings of aging has shown that in many model organisms, the rate of aging can be controlled by altering conserved signaling pathways and processes, implying that the aging process itself may ultimately be receptive to therapeutic manipulation.

Dietary restriction and aging (intermittent fasting)

Dietary restriction, defined as the restriction of nutrients while avoiding malnutrition, is the most effective way of reducing aging. Dietary restriction was first observed to delay aging and disease in lab rats about a century ago. Since then, the effects of dietary restriction on aging has been studied greatly. Dietary restriction has been observed to extend the lifespan of yeast, invertebrates, fish, dogs, hamsters, mice and apes. Different molecular mechanisms have been proposed to improve the positive effects of dietary restriction on longevity, including insulin/IGF-1 and TOR signaling. However, it is currently unknown to what level lifespan extension resulting from dietary reduction is mediated by these nutrient-sensing pathways.

Aging (summary)

Aging results from the gradual decline in cellular repair and body mechanisms, which leads to an accumulation of unwanted cellular constituents and ultimately leads to the degeneration of tissues and organs. Decades of research have shown that the aging process is influenced by genetics and that many metabolic genes can influence aging by mechanisms still to be fully elucidated. Autophagy promotes cell maintenance by removing unwanted materials and by using recycled components as an alternative nutrient resource. This shows that autophagy aids longevity because an organism can recover more effectively from stress-induced cellular damage. Evidence that autophagy influences the aging process has been observed in different organisms, from yeast to multicellular organisms such as worms and flies.

CHAPTER SEVEN: Autophagic Lifestyle

Autophagic meal plan

An autophagy-based lifestyle is key to living a healthy life and avoiding complications. Following an autophagy meal plan can help make sure that a person is getting their daily nutritional needs. It also gives you more options and can help in weight loss. We will now concentrate on autophagy meal plans.

We have done justice to exercise and fasting, but an autophagy meal plan can help an individual keep track of carbs and calories and make healthy eating more interesting by introducing some new ideas to the diet. No one plan will suit everyone. Each individual should work out their own meal plan with help from a doctor or dietitian.

Steps to take in creating an autophagy meal plan

- Balancing carbohydrate intake with activity levels and the use of insulin and other medications.
- Substituting calories with plenty of fiber to help manage blood sugar levels and reduce the risk of high cholesterol, weight gain, cardiovascular disease and other health issues.
- Reducing intake of processed carbohydrates and foods with added sugars (e.g. rice, spaghetti, cookies, etc.) which are more likely to cause a high sugar peak than whole grains and vegetables. • Studying and understanding how dietary choices can impact your health (e.g. the fact that salt increases the risk of high blood pressure). • Reducing and managing weight, as this can help a person manage the development of diseases and complications.
- Taking into account individual treatment plans, which will contain recommendations from a doctor or dietitian.

Key points to note

- Having the right food measurement can help an individual monitor his or her food consumption more accurately.
- You can still enjoy a healthy, diverse diet that helps your body stay nourished.

As we noted earlier, this involves carefully:

- Balancing food consumption in order to meet the specific diet requirements,

- Getting appropriate measurement of portions,
- Creating meal plans.

Other factors to note when setting up a meal guide

- Take into account the daily consumption of carbs and calories. Take
- your time to determine the quantity of carbs that would meet your required daily consumption.
- Divide the quantity between the meals for the day.
- Always try to treat yourself. This can be done by doing a checklist of your favorite meals and including them in your dishes with respect to the carb requirements.
- Use resources available to you to fill out your daily meal schedule.
- Take note of your blood sugar levels to monitor the rate of results your meal guide is yielding.

Autophagy meal planning methods

These are some diabetes meal planning methods. Each has its peculiarities. It all depends on your targets or the state of your health.

Weight Management Method

There is without a doubt a link between diseases and body weight (obesity). Many people suffering from a disease may be aiming to lose weight or prevent weight gain. One method of achieving this is by "counting calories". The number of calories that a person needs each day will depend on factors such as: blood glucose targets, activity levels, height, sex, specific plans to lose, gain or maintain weight, the use of insulin and other medications, preferences, budget.

Dash Method

The DASH method is made up of the DASH diet, which focuses mainly on fruits, vegetables, whole grains, nuts and seeds. Other components include dairy products, poultry and fish that are low in fat or totally fat-free. This encourages people to avoid added salt, sugars, unhealthy fats, red meats and processed carbs. The dash diet has two targets: to reduce blood pressure levels and to help individuals lose weight and become fit.

Plate method

This method is growing in popularity. The plate method can help an individual get the right amount of each type of food. Getting the right nutritional contents/value from diets is important for everyone. The plate method uses the image of a standard 9-inch dinner plate to help people visualize nutritional balance as they plan their meals. It basically involves dividing your plate into sections, half (50%) for vegetables and fruits with the remaining half for protein, fat and carbohydrates. This more than meets the current recommended guidelines.

Carbohydrate swapping method

Although not a popular method, it is one way to manage blood sugar levels. You simply have to decide how many carbohydrates to consume each day and how to divide them between meals. You then create a replacement chart where you replace normal day-to-day carbohydrates (unhealthy carbs) with healthy ones. The carbohydrate chart ranks foods according to the number of carbs they contain, making it simpler to swap one type of food for another.

As always, seek advice from seasoned professionals. They might adjust your meal plan to suit your specific needs.

The Glycemic Index Method

The glycemic index (GI) ranks foods according to how quickly they raise blood sugar levels. Foods with high sugar loads increase blood sugar levels rapidly. Examples include sugars and other highly processed carbs. Foods with low scores contain none or few carbs, or they contain fiber, which the body does not absorb as quickly as processed carbs.

Listed below are some examples of carbohydrate-rich foods and their GI scores:

Foods considered low GI (having scores less than 55): pure stone-ground bread (especially pure wheat), unpeeled sweet potatoes and oats.

Benefits of an Autophagy Meal Plan

For clarification purposes we will briefly highlight the benefits of having an autophagy meal plan.

It helps save money

Meal planning helps you save money because you will know ahead of time what you will be cooking, and you will already have your grocery list ready to go. You will be able to plan meals around items you already have at home, which means you won't overspend on groceries, some of which will end up going bad and ultimately being tossed – the result of not following a list and buying too much. With meal planning, you buy what you need.

Knowing ahead of time what you will be cooking for the week will also save you from eating out and ordering fast-food. This doesn't only pertain to dinnertime. When you plan your meals and make sure to include leftovers for lunch, you will also save hundreds of dollars every month by not buying food near work.

Waste less time

An individual suffering from a disease may spend a lot of time on cooking homemade meals. More often than not, time is not only wasted on the cooking itself, but also while thinking about what to cook, making the grocery list and shopping for items. If you plan ahead to cook freezerfriendly meals in bulk, you will be able to save trips to the grocery store and time during busy weeknights. Saving time in the present is just as important as saving time in the future.

Waste Less

Statistics show that the average American throws away about 300 dollars' worth of food every year. Saving that money is a much better option. There is nothing more annoying than seeing food you bought with your hardearned money wasted. By planning out all the meals you will be cooking, you ensure that no food gets wasted. As you prepare your meals, you will find this very rewarding and fulfilling.

Stress less

One of the most stressful aspects of daily living is planning meals. Thinking about these meals on a daily basis can be very frustrating. That is why having a meal plan in place can stop this unnecessary stress and allow you to slip easily into cooking time.

With an autophagy meal plan, you can expect to lower your stress levels. After following a meal plan, you gradually learn on the rope and you might soon find yourself making a new one in the future.

Lose weight (reduce sugar levels)

Home-cooked meals are healthier than eating out, because cooking at home gives you complete control over what you put into your body. Foods made in restaurants are great to indulge once in a while, but they are laden with sugar, sodium and fat. These are detrimental to the health of any diabetes sufferer.

But cooking in itself is not always easy. It is the meal planning part that keeps you motivated to continue cooking and stick to eating healthier. When you stick to a meal plan and enjoy more home-cooked meals, your body will start seeing results, whether you lose weight or feel physically and emotionally good overall.

Creates more options

An autophagy meal plan exposes you to a wider variety of healthy foods. This helps you have your cake and eat it. You stay healthy while eating delicious meals. In fact, if you don't plan meals, you are actually more likely to eat the same meals. This is simple logic. If you are familiar with making spaghetti and meat-stew, chances are you are going to make them over and over again to save time from thinking about what else to prepare. This could become very boring.

However, when planning meals, you can include new recipes. After all, they say that variety is the spice of life.

Learn portion control

Planning your own meals will allow you to see how much you are actually eating. This also prevents you from overeating at restaurants, which tend to serve a way bigger portion than you should actually be eating.

Eat healthy

When you are hungry and your blood sugar drops, you are more inclined to eat whatever you can get your hands on the fastest. This is why some of us settle for the closest fast-food joint with unhealthy options. Meal planning eliminates this issue when you have a balanced meal at your fingertips, filled with nutrient-dense food prepped and ready to go!

Many times, unhealthy foods are chosen because of convenience. Therefore, having an autophagy meal plan is a no brainer. *It is your gateway to staying healthy and enjoying your life.*

Meals that help you achieve autophagy

Vegetable omelets

Veggie omelets are filled with protein and fiber. All of the ingredients, from spices to eggs and veggies, are filled with a lot of nutrients, including lots of proteins and fiber. Its high fiber content makes it filling and satisfying. Vegetables are one of the healthiest ways to fuel the body for a morning full of productivity.

Ingredients:

- 1 teaspoon olive or coconut oil
- 1 tablespoon red bell pepper (shredded)
- 1 tablespoon sliced or chopped onion
- 1/4 cup sliced mushrooms
- Fresh spinach leaves
- 2 eggs (beaten)
- Water
- Pepper

Preparation:

- Using an 8-inch nonstick skillet, gently heat oil over medium heat. Add the pepper, onion and mushrooms at once. Cook for about 3 minutes, stirring frequently, until onion is soft. Add the spinach and stir. Continue cooking and stirring until the spinach becomes tender. Transfer the vegetables from the pan to a plate.
- In small bowl, beat the eggs together with water, salt and pepper with a fork or whisk until they form a smooth consistency. Reheat the skillet over medium heat. Quickly pour the egg mixture into the pan. Slide the pan back and forth rapidly over medium heat, stir with a wooden spoon to spread the eggs uniformly over the bottom of the pan as it hardens. Let it sit over mild heat for 30 seconds to lightly brown the bottom of the omelet. Try not to overcook. The omelet will continue to cook after folding.

Place the cooked vegetable mixture on one side of the omelet. Add cheese (optional) with a wooden spoon, fold the remaining half of the omelet over the vegetables. Gently slide out the mixture into your serving plate. Serve immediately.

Servings: 1

Nutritional values per serving:

Calories: 172 Kcal

Fat: 15.2 g

Carbohydrates: 5.7 g

Dietary Fiber: 1.7 g

Sugar: 3.4 g

Protein: 13.5 g

Ingredient Nutritional Analysis:

Olive oil

Olive oil protects the body against cognitive decline. Recent research has shown that the consumption of olive oil protects the brain and our learning ability.

It prevents the formation of amyloid-beta plaques in the brain. This is a classic marker of most neuro-degenerative diseases.

Olive oil prevents brain inflammation, but most importantly activates autophagy.

Harvested brain cells from rats fed on diets enriched with olive oil had increased levels of autophagy and reduced amyloidosis.

- It is believed that olive oil is better than fruits and vegetables alone, and as an unsaturated vegetable fat it is healthier than saturated animal fats.

Researchers believe that an olive oil enriched diet improves working memory, spatial memory and learning abilities.

Olive oil increases autophagy activation, which can help reduce levels of amyloidosis.

This could be revolutionary. Autophagy activation in the brain will improve memory and synaptic integrity, and it can equally prevent the development of Alzheimer's disease.

Coconut oil

Though butter would make this dish tastier, coconut oil contains much less of both cholesterol and sodium than butter. This makes it healthier. Although coconut oil contains more calories, when used in little amounts, these calories are negligible.

Coconuts are high in naturally occurring unsaturated fat from short and long chain fatty acids.

These fatty acid chains are converted in the body into monolaurin, a useful compound that destroys a wide variety of pathogens. It helps fight common colds and viral infections, such as the flu.

Coconuts also contain the following essential nutrients that have tremendous benefits for the cell/tissue/body:

- Vitamin C
- Thiamin (vitamin B1)
- Folate
- Potassium
- Manganese
- Copper
- Selenium
- Iron
- Phosphorous
- Potassium

Coconut can be consumed in many different ways, and it can have numerous benefits for people with compromised immune systems and diabetes.

Coconut oil has recognized health properties when applied on the skin, but it can also have benefits when used in a diet.

Coconut oil should be used with caution. It has about 19 per cent more calories than the same amount of butter.

Coconut milk

Coconut milk is obtained from the coconut flesh. Coconut milk can come in two main forms:

- A thick form, called coco cream, that is used in rich sauces.
- A more fluid form, containing more water, that can be used instead of milk.

The more fluid form of coconut milk has the same number of calories as semi-skimmed milk. However, there are more calories in the thicker form (coco cream) and caution needs to be exercised in regard to portion sizes.

Coconut flour

- Coconut flour is rich in fiber, which can prevent the risk of developing heart disease and can lower cholesterol levels.

It is low in dietary sugar compared to flours such as wheat. It is useful for people with diabetes as it helps them reduce blood glucose levels.

It is gluten free. This makes it a good option for people with celiac disease – an autoimmune disease that diabetes sufferers are more at risk of developing.

Additionally, coconut flour is a good source of protein, which keeps you full for longer and is valuable for cell regeneration (autophagy).

Coconut water

Coconut water is often regarded as the perfect hangover cure as it is naturally refreshing and full of minerals that can prevent nausea and/or vomiting.

Coconut water is the clear fluid found in young coconuts. It consists mostly of water. It contains very little fat and is very low in calories.

Eggs

The eggs account for almost all the cholesterol and sodium in the meal, but their cholesterol is the healthy type. It originates from Omega-3 fatty acids (especially fresh ones straight from the poultry). Eggs are also heavily responsible for making the meal filling. Eggs have been relied upon as a source of breakfast nutrients for centuries.

Vegetables and spices

The remaining ingredients in this omelet carry most of the nutrients in the meal (the seasoning and the vegetables). They contain lots of vitamin A and C, calcium and iron. The peppers contain most of the vitamin C. The spinach adds the potassium and is also a rich source of iron.

Yogurt breakfast pudding

Ingredients:

- 5-ounce bowl containing vanilla yogurt, one with considerably low fat
- 1/2 cup oats, go for the rolled ones
- A glass of milk
- 1/2 glass blended pineapple (juice pack)
- 2 teaspoons chia seeds
- 1/2 tablespoon fine vanilla
- 1/2 teaspoon cinnamon, preferably blended

3 tablespoons grated almonds

- Red apple properly chopped in fine pieces *Preparation:*

Get a moderately sized bowl, pour in the yogurt, add the rolled oats, blended pineapple, half of glass of milk, teaspoons of chia seeds, fine vanilla and blended cinnamon. Stir well and pour into a container with a good lid. Cover appropriately and place in the refrigerator. Your content is perfect for consumption after a few hours.

Stir well before serving. Serve chilled. You can lace each serving with a spoon of almonds (optional).

Servings: 2

Nutritional values per serving:

Calories: 325 Kcal

Fat:10.6g

Carbohydrates: 44.5g

Dietary Fiber: 7.6g

Sugar: 26.2g

- Protein: 13.6g

Ingredient Nutritional Analysis:

Yogurt

Yogurt is without a doubt a great nutrient-dense breakfast option. If unsweetened (natural/without sugar), it is low in sugar and high in protein. This implies that it would not cause blood sugar to increase.

Fermented foods like yogurt contain good bacteria called probiotics. Probiotics help improve gut health. Although research on gut health is elementary, gut bacteria contributes greatly to the overall health of the body and can help resolve a number of health conditions, including obesity and high blood pressure.

Ongoing research shows that yogurt consumption might be associated with lower levels of glucose and insulin resistance in the body, together with lower systolic blood pressure. Nutritional analysis shows that yogurt, when included in a diet, can reduce the risk of type 2 diabetes in healthy and older adults. Another quality yogurt possesses is its low Glycemic Index (GI).

Yogurt and autophagy

High-fat diets cause obesity, leading to heart disease and autophagy imbalance.

Recent research showed the amazing effects of probiotics on high-fat induced obesity, heart disease and autophagy in the hearts of mice. Sevenweek-old male mice were separated randomly into three equally sized experimental groups, namely normal diet and high-fat diet groups. Mice fed with a high-fat diet augmented with low to medium or increased doses of probiotic powders. These experiments were set up for a 9-week trial period. The structure of the left ventricle was analyzed using Masson's trichrome staining and immunohistochemistry staining. Key probiotics-related pathway substances were evaluated using western blotting. Abnormal myocardial structure and enlarged interstitial spaces were seen in HF hearts. These interstitial spaces were greatly reduced in mice provided with probiotics (yogurt) compared with HF hearts. HF was increased after probiotic supplementation was significantly decreased. This research has shown that oral administration of yogurt may prevent heart disease and cardiac hypertrophy. It also shows that yogurt aids the autophagy-signaling pathway in obese rats. These experiments are almost 100% bound to create the same effects in humans.

Coconut Berry Sunrise Smoothies

Smoothies are rich in nutrients. They contain a lot of fruits and vegetables. A smoothie can be a good way to consume a rich variety of foods. As mentioned before, these foods include fruits, vegetables and even fat, proteins and many others.

How to make a great smoothie:

-*Include healthful fats:* there are many good sources of healthful fats that can be used in smoothies, such as fats from avocado and chia seeds. Healthful fats can be good for the body. Fats play an important role in the body, and they can help reduce the speed at which sugar enters the blood. Thus, they can help reduce hunger or its onset. Examples of healthy fat sources are almond and peanut butter, chia seeds, avocado, raw pecans and raw walnuts. *It should be noted that no matter how healthy fats might seem, they should be taken in reasonable amounts.*

-*Top up with protein*: in a similar way as fat, protein offers many health benefits that are essential for the body. High-protein content helps to slow the absorption of food, and this reduces the rate at which sugar enters the bloodstream. Protein can be animal or vegetable based. Vegetable based proteins are healthier. Adding high-protein ingredients to a smoothie can offer tremendous health benefits. Suitable proteins for smoothies include: plain unsweetened Greek yogurt, hemp and other seeds, almonds, pea protein and whey protein.

Furthermore, adding leafy greens like spinach can increase your smoothie's nutritional value.

-*Include fiber*: fiber can be soluble or insoluble. Insoluble fiber is harder. It takes the body more time to break down soluble fiber. Fiber takes longer to release its energy, reducing the risk of a glucose spike. Insoluble fiber boosts digestion and reduces the absorption of other foods in the gastrointestinal tract. Fiber creates satiety. These attributes can benefit a person with diabetes by reducing the risks of a blood sugar spike, an increase in cholesterol and weight gain. Through these ways, fiber can lower the chance of various complications related to most diseases, high blood sugar and many other health conditions. High-fiber foods that can be included in a smoothie are: raspberries, oranges, nectarines, peaches and blueberries and vegetables such as spinach, grinded nuts (kale nuts) and seeds (chia seeds).

-Reduce Sugar: many foods used in preparing smoothies already have sugar in them. Processed foods often contain added sugar. Avoid using sugar (try to keep things as natural as possible). When choosing ingredients, take note of the following: honey and maple syrup contain reasonable amounts of sugar, ripe fruits contain more sugar than less ripe ones and milk contains lactose which is also a form of sugar. Spices are not exempted either. Spices such as cinnamon, nutmeg, ginger or turmeric fruits can be used in smoothies. Turmeric contains a natural source of sugar, as well as fiber. It is better to sweeten smoothies with natural ingredients rather than adding sugar/sweeteners. They are not good for the body.

-Reduce carbohydrate content: w hen making a smoothie, try to make sure you know the quantity of carbohydrates you are adding. Researchers recommend that people should look to include 45 grams or less of carbohydrates in a smoothie. Some examples of carbohydrates that can be added to smoothies are: banana, melon, blueberries, plain yogurt and granola. A healthy smoothie should contain spinach or other dark leafy vegetables. These contain fewer carbohydrates per serving and offer healthy nutritional benefits.

Using measuring cups, spoons and the diabetes exchange list is a good way to measure the quantity of carbohydrates to put in the smoothie. A medical professional (doctor/dietician) will advise on how many carbs a person should consume each day and at each meal. This will vary between individuals based on their height, weight, activity levels and medications.

About coconut berry sunrise smoothies

A rich blend of strawberries and blueberries gives this smoothie a vibrant purplish color. Coconut water, dairy-free vanilla yogurt and hemp seeds add a touch of nutty sweetness to give this smoothie bowl a refreshing natural taste.

Ingredients:

- 1 cup coconut water
- 1 cup coconut yogurt, vanilla flavored
- 2/3 cup fresh or frozen strawberries
- 1/2 cup fresh or slightly chilled blueberries
- 3 tablespoons hemp seeds or 2 tablespoons vanilla protein powder

Extra Ingredients:

- Sunrise Crunchy Cereal
- Dried coconut
- Fresh blackberries
- Cherries
- Blueberries

Preparation:

- First, prepare the toppings for the smoothie bowl. Add dried coconut, fresh blackberries, cherries and blueberries to top this berry coconut smoothie bowl.
- In a highspeed blender, add coconut water, dairy-free yogurt, frozen berries and hemp seeds. Blend on high until it has a fine texture. Shake the blender at intervals to ensure the mixture blends well (becomes homogeneous).
- Pour the smoothie into a bowl and add the toppings (optional).

Notes:

Use frozen berries if you want a thick, frosty smoothie bowl. Choose fresh fruit if you desire a thinner consistency.

To get a different flavor, you can substitute the coconut water for vanilla almond milk.

Servings: 2

Nutritional values per serving:

Calories: 148 Kcal

Fat: 7.5g

Carbohydrates: 17.8g

Dietary Fiber: 5.6g

Sugar: 10.2g

Protein: 4.9g

Ingredient Nutritional Analysis:

Berries

Adding more richness to your diet in the form of berries is encouraged by many nutritionists. The amazing effect of berries against inflammation has been documented in many researches. Diets augmented with blueberries and strawberries have also been shown to increase behavior and cognitive functions in stressed young rats.

To analyze the amazing effects of berries on brain activity, specifically the ability of the brain to clear toxic waste, researchers fed mice a berry diet for 3 months and then studied their brains after irradiation. All the mice were fed berries 2 months before radiation and then divided into two groups. The mice in one group were evaluated after one and a half day of radiation and the others after 30 days.

After 30 days on berry diet, the rats experienced substantial protection from radiation compared to control.

The researchers studied neurochemical changes in the brain, particularly what is known as autophagy. Autophagy can regulate the synthesis, degradation and recycling of cellular components in the brain. It also helps the brain clear toxic wastes. Most brain disorders such as Alzheimer's and Parkinson's have shown an increased amount of toxic accumulation. Berries promote autophagy, the brain's natural maintenance mechanism, thereby reducing the toxic wastes.

Sweet potato, onion and turkey sausage hash

Sweet potato and turkey sausage hash is a great option for breakfast. It is gluten and dairy free. It is one of those few meals you can have for both breakfast and lunch. It is very easy to make and doesn't involve much processing.

Ingredients:

- 1/2 pound of turkey sausage hash
- 1 cup onion sliced
- 1/2 cup red bell pepper sliced
- 3 cups sweet potato sliced
- 1/4 tablespoon salt
- 1/4 teaspoon ground black pepper
- 1/4 teaspoon cinnamon
- 1/8 tablespoon cumin
- 1/8 teaspoon chili powder

Preparation:

- Preheat a skillet over low heat.
- Add the sausage to the pan. Break it up into small clumps.
- Cook for about 6 minutes. Stop when the sausage turns brown. Remove the sausage from the skillet and place it on a plate.
- Spray the skillet with a cooking spray and add the onion, bell pepper, sweet potato, salt, pepper, cinnamon, cumin and chili powder all at once. Stir until you achieve a good consistency.
- Cook for another 5-8 minutes, stirring occasionally, until the sweet potatoes become soft.
- Add in the sausage and stir to combine.
- Finally, cook without stirring for 5 minutes. Serve hot.

Serving: 4

Nutritional values per serving:

Calories: 250 Kcal

Fat: 3.2g

Carbohydrates: 35.2g

Dietary Fiber: 6g

Sugar: 11.7g

Protein: 20.2g

Ingredient Nutritional Analysis:

Sweet potatoes

The sweet potato is gaining increased attention today, thanks in part to its low glycemic index (GI) rating. Sweet potatoes are ranked lower than white potatoes on the GI and they can help people with diabetes better manage their blood sugar levels.

Sweet potatoes are very rich in vitamins, including vitamin A which helps to keep the eyes healthy, vitamin C which helps the human immune system, iron which helps red blood cells to make oxygen and transport nutrients throughout the body. They are a great source of fiber, which can also stimulate the feeling of fullness. Even the roots of sweet potatoes are nutritious, although they are not frequently used in human diets/meals (they are used mostly in food for animals).

However, it should be noted that sweet potatoes are still carbohydrates and should be consumed in reduced quantities. Studies on rats (food and function research 2014) have proven that sweet potatoes help reduce high blood pressure, increase cardiovascular function while simultaneously supplying the body with antioxidants.

Ask a medical professional (dietician/doctor) for advice, as your health status may require a different approach.

Sweet potatoes and autophagy

Sweet potatoes are known to suppress endothelial senescence as well as to bring back cellular function in test rats. Researchers discovered that sweet potatoes aided autophagy to prevent that an increased level of glucose undoes endothelial senescence. Also, sweet potatoes prevented the prospects of endothelium getting older in rats with diabetes through the increase of autophagy. Reduction in autophagy led to a higher endothelial senescence, whereas increase in autophagy led to a lower level of senescence. In summary, sweet potatoes increased cellular autophagy, later on attenuated NLRP3 actions and also prevented endothelial senescence thereby reducing cardiovascular complications.

Sweet potatoes delay endothelial senescence by increasing autophagy!

Crispy breakfast pita with eggs

This very delicious meal is very light but surprisingly filling. It is easy to prepare and is a good option to consider when you want a quickie.

Ingredients:

- 6-8 slices of pita breads
- Olive oil
- 6 large eggs
- 3/4 cup mascarpone cheese
- Sliced zest of 1/2 large lemon
- Salt
- Freshly ground black pepper
- 3 tablespoons fresh lemon juice
- 3 packed cups arugula or baby spinach
- 8 oz thinly sliced prosciutto

Preparation:

- Gently heat a grill pan over medium-high heat. Brush each side of your pita breads with 1/2 teaspoon olive oil and grill for about 2-3 minutes on each side, until they become crispy. Remove from the grill and cool slightly.

- In a large skillet, heat 1 tablespoon of olive oil over low-medium heat. Crack the eggs directly into the pan and cook until the egg whites form (2-3 minutes).

- Mix the mascarpone cheese, lemon zest, 1/2 teaspoon salt and 1/2 teaspoon pepper in a small bowl.
- In another bowl (medium size) whisk together 3 tablespoons olive oil, the lemon juice, 1 teaspoon salt and 1/2 tablespoon of pepper until smooth. Add the arugula and toss until coated.
- Spread each pita with 2 tablespoons of the mascarpone mixture. Divide the prosciutto into two (on top). Do the same to the arugula and place it on top of the prosciutto. Tactfully place a fried egg on top of each pita. Sprinkle the eggs with a pinch of salt and pepper and serve.

Servings: 6

Nutritional values per serving:

Calories: 391 Kcal

Fat: 16.6g

Carbohydrates: 36.3g

Dietary Fiber: 1.7g

Sugar: 1.7g

Protein: 23.5g

Ingredient Nutritional Analysis:

Eggs

Eggs are very nutritious. One large egg contains about half of gram of carbohydrates, which means you can avoid adding a lot of unnecessary sugar.

A full egg contains about 7 grams of protein. Eggs are equally rich in potassium, which helps to support nerve and muscle health. Potassium balances the effect of sodium in the body. Eggs equally promote the cardiovascular functions of the heart.

- Furthermore, eggs have other healthy nutrients, such as lutein and
- choline, vitamin A (egg yolk) and calcium. Lutein protects you against disease, and choline improves the functioning of the brain. Egg yolks contain biotin, which is important for healthy hair, skin and nails (appendages), as well as insulin production. Eggs from pastured chickens are high in omega-3s, which are beneficial fats for people with diabetes.

Eggs contribute little to body fat. One large egg has only about 75 calories and 5 grams of fat, of which only a mere 1.6 grams are saturated fats. Eggs are complete meal agents and can be prepared in different ways to suit your tastes. They can be combined with a lot of foods to great effects (e.g. tomatoes, spinach or other vegetables). Although eggs are very healthy, they should be eaten with moderation.

Generally, one should limit egg consumption to three a week. If you only eat the egg whites, you can eat a little more (about 5). If you must fry your eggs, make sure you use unsaturated oils.

Boiled egg is a good high-protein snack. The protein will help keep you satisfied without affecting your blood sugar. Protein not only slows digestion, but it equally reduces glucose absorption. This is very helpful for the body.

Crustless spinach and mushroom quiche

Ingredients:

- 1 tablespoon of olive oil
- 1 tablespoon of butter
- 1 lb fresh spinach leaves
- 1/4 cup yellow onion, chopped
- 2 cloves garlic minced
- 10 eggs (briskly mixed with a fork)
- 8 oz cremini mushrooms, rough chopped, stems removed
-
-

3 oz feta cheese crumbled Salt

and pepper to taste *Preparation:*

Heat your oven to about 350°F.
Roast the mushrooms by gradually tossing them with olive oil. Season with salt and pepper (little) to taste.

- Spread the mushrooms on a baking sheet and allow to roast for about 25-30 minutes. Allow to cool enough, after which you chop.
- In a medium sized skillet, dissolve the butter on low to medium heat.
- Add your spinach and cook until it to begins to wilt.
- Add the onion, then continue cooking, stirring periodically (every 1 minute) until the spinach is wilted and the onion has softened (3-5 minutes).
- Add the garlic, then stir on low heat for about 1-2 minutes.
- Remove from heat, then mix in the eggs, distributing the spinach and mushrooms evenly.
- Pour into your prepared quiche dish and sprinkle with feta cheese.
- Bake for 20 minutes or until set. Serve warm (steamy).

Servings: 6

Nutritional values per serving:

Calories: 210 Kcal

Fat: 14.9g

Carbohydrates: 6.2g

Dietary Fiber: 2g

Sugar: 2.3g

Protein: 14.5g

Ingredient Nutritional Analysis:

- *Mushrooms*
-

Mushrooms contribute greatly to the body. They supply it with vital nutrients, can reduce/subside inflammation and are anti-cancerous. Here are some reasons mushrooms should be added to your diet.

They have anticancer and antiviral properties that have been used in Asia since the olden times. Mushrooms have immune properties and have recently been used in HIV treatment. They equally help reduce blood pressure.

Mushrooms help reduce body cholesterol, fight infections, reduce menopausal symptoms and fatigue.

Some species of mushrooms display anti-oxidative properties, reduce DNA damage, aid eyesight, fight colds, viral infections, reduce blood sugar (diabetes treatment) and much more.

Mushrooms and autophagy

Mushrooms induce autophagy in body cells to promote cell death. In a recent research, SUM-149 cells were treated with 1.0 mg/mL of mushrooms for 2h, 4h, 6h, 8h, 12h and 24h. To analyze autophagy effects on cell viability, cells were treated with 3-methyladenine (3-MA), chloroquine and PP242 with or without mushrooms for 1 day. Results showed that mushrooms affect the expression of autophagy-related molecules depending on treatment time. Mushrooms increase the expression of autophagy proteins in body cells. Additionally, the autophagy inhibitors heightened cell viability after one day, while cancer cell viability decreased when mushrooms were added.

Thus, mushrooms induce autophagy, promoting cell death in body cells, as cancer cell viability is decreased, with an increase in pro-apoptotic protein expression when they are added in.

Lamb Stew

This is a very rich and delicious meal. You may be tempted to reserve it for special occasions. It is a household favorite. It has a rich protein content which makes it suitable for growing children and adolescents. Although its suitability cuts across age and growth needs, the lamb stew recipe is growing in popularity around the world.

Ingredients:

2 oz chopped bacon
3 oz lamb

- 1 tablespoon salt
- A handful of flour
- 1 bulb onion
- 1/2 teaspoon ground garlic
- 1 tablespoon tomato paste
- 1/2 teaspoon pepper
- 1/2 teaspoon dried thyme
- 2 bay leaves
- 3 oz nearly sliced potatoes
- 2 oz well grated carrot
- 1oz of thickly sliced mushrooms

2 cups vegetable stock *Preparation:*

- In a large pot, heat the chopped bacon over medium heat until it becomes golden brown and the fat is released. Transfer the bacon with a slotted spoon to a large plate.
- While the bacon cooks, season your sliced lamb meat with 1/2 tablespoon of salt, pepper and 1/2 onion. Sprinkle the flour around the meat (1/4). Mix the flour and meat together. Cook the lamb under mild heat, and bacon grease over mild heat until it becomes brown (3-4 minutes per side), after which you place it together with the bacon. • Add sliced onion and heat gently for 2 minutes. Add garlic and heat gently for another minute, stirring constantly. Add thickly sliced mushrooms, bring to a simmer and cook 10 minutes uncovered.

Preheat the oven at 325°F.

- • Return the bacon and lamb back to the pot then add 2 cups of broth, 1
- tablespoon tomato paste, 1 teaspoon salt, 1/2 teaspoon pepper, 1/2 teaspoon dried thyme and 2 bay leaves. Add the potatoes and carrots then stir to combine (potatoes should be mostly submerged in liquid). Bring to a boil then cover with a lid and carefully transfer into the preheated oven at 325˚F for 1 hour and 45 minutes. When cooked, potatoes will be easy to pierce, and the lamb will be very tender. To reduce fat content, spoon out any excess oil at the surface of the stew.

- Serve with sugar free bread to soak up that broth which is loaded with amazing goodies.

Servings: 2

Nutritional values per serving:

Calories: 371 Kcal

Fat: 17.5g

Carbohydrates: 31.1g

Dietary Fiber: 5.6g

Sugar: 7.5g

Protein: 27g

Ingredient Nutritional Analysis:

Onions

Quercetin, a flavonoid found in onions, was reported to effectively inhibit 2-amino-1-methyl-6-phenylimidazo[4, 5-b]pyridine (PhIP) in food. Quercetin is converted into a novel compound 8-C-(Ephenylethenyl)quercetin(8-CEPQ). This compound can help prevent cancer. It is also known to promote autophagy.

Mozzarella and artichoke sauce

Although often considered a vegetable, artichokes are actually a type of thistle.

Ingredients:

- 3 oz mozzarella
- 2 oz artichoke
-

- 1 bulb of onions
- 1 tablespoon pepper
  1/2 lb meat (preferably chicken) or fish
- A plate of chopped tomatoes
- A pinch of spices of choice

Preparation:

- Fry the tomatoes with olive oil (add pepper, onions, spices of choice), preboil chicken with your spices of choice, pepper and salt. Mix everything together and after about 3 minutes add the artichokes and mozzarella. Serve warm or hot.

Servings: 2

Nutritional values per serving:

Calories: 328 Kcal

Fat: 13.6g

Carbohydrates: 15.4g

Dietary Fiber: 5.9g

Sugar: 4g

Protein: 38.3g

Ingredient Nutritional Analysis :

Artichokes

Artichokes are the real deal. They are low in fat while rich in fiber, vitamins, minerals and antioxidants. They are equally high in folate and vitamins C and K. They are also rich in important minerals such as magnesium, phosphorus, potassium and iron. To cap it all, they are rich in antioxidants as well.

Artichokes and autophagy

This vegetable has several benefits for our body. Artichokes contain inulin, a carbohydrate that is metabolized very slowly in our body, which is suitable for diabetics. Artichokes are very rich in fiber, and therefore help reduce blood sugar and control cholesterol levels. In addition, this vegetable can combat constipation.

The artichoke also contains cynarin. Cynarin stimulates bile secretion. Bile favors the digestion of fats and stops the retention of liquids (diuretic effect). The artichoke's caloric content is very low. It has less than 1% fat, and this is about 22 calories per 100 grams. Therefore, the weight loss ability of the artichoke is due to three reasons: its low-calorie content, its diuretic effect and its ability to digest fats and eliminate them. This makes artichokes very effective in respect to autophagy.

In addition to all that was listed, artichokes improve liver function as it works as a cleanser of the intestines, liver and kidneys.

Lower weight with artichoke water: artichoke water can be consumed three times a day. and at least 10 times a month. It can be used to treat obesity and also detoxify the body.

Herbed butter

Butter is classified under fats and oil. It is very beneficial for autophagy. Herbed butter not only stimulates autophagy, but it also contains nutrient rich herbs that stimulate the human immune system.

Ingredients:

You can make and prepare herbed butter out of any combination of your favorite herbs:

- Cream the butter and herbs together and season with salt and pepper.
-

Preparation:

- On a sheet of waxed paper, massage the butter into a log and roll up tightly. Fold the end flaps over to seal the butter.

  Freeze. When set, slice off 1" pieces as needed and close the end. Prepare ahead of time and freeze your butter, so it will be ready to go when you desire.

Serving size: 30g

Nutritional values per serving:

Calories: 210 Kcal

Fat: 23g

Protein: 0,3g

Carbohydrates: 0g

Fiber: 0g

Ingredient Nutritional Analysis:

Butter

Butter has long been a cause of controversy in the world of nutrition. Many nutritionists believe it increases cholesterol levels and clogs the arteries, while others think it can be a nutritious and flavorful addition to the diet. Fortunately, a lot of research has been conducted in recent years evaluating the potential health effects of butter. Recent research has shown that many of the old beliefs were wrong. Butter has a rich flavor and creamy texture. Although butter is high in calories and fat, it contains some very important nutrients. For example, butter is a good source of vitamin A, a soluble vitamin needed for good eyesight, smooth skin and immune function. It contains vitamin E, which improves heart health and serves as an antioxidant to protect the body against damage caused by molecules called free radicals. Butter also contains very small amounts of other nutrients. Examples include riboflavin, niacin, calcium, and phosphorus. It has a high calorie content. This means a very small quantity can provide the body with lots of energy. The idea behind using butter for weight loss is that by eating reduced amounts, you can induce weight loss through ketogenesis, one of the pillars of autophagy.

Pork carnitas

Ingredients:

- 2 tablespoons groundnut oil
- 2 kg of pork, cut into several large pieces
- 2 tablespoons salt
- 2 onions, chopped
- 1 clove garlic, crushed
- 4 teaspoons blended and already juiced lime
- 2 teaspoons finely blended chili
- A pinch of blended dry oregano
- 1 tablespoon blended cumin
- 14.5 oz chicken broth

Preparation:

- Make the groundnut really hot, in an oven over low heat. Sprinkle your pork with a little salt and seasoning, then place the pork in the oven. Cook for about 5 minutes. Add all the other ingredients except the chicken broth. Incorporate your chicken broth after a little while and boil. Reduce the heat in the oven, safely place the cover and occasionally stir until your pork becomes tender. This will take about 1 hour.
- After this, allow the oven to heat up until at least 300°F.
-

- Move your pork to an already spread sheet. Do not throw away the
- liquid resulted from boiling your pork. Lace the pork in some of this liquid and add sauce to the mix.
- Bake your pork until it becomes brown in the already heated up oven, normally a little over 20 minutes. Spray a little more liquid saved from before on the pork, every 5 minutes. Slice the meat as it turns brown.
- Serve hot.

Servings: 8

Nutritional values per serving:

Calories: 440 Kcal

Fat: 13.5g

Carbohydrates: 5.8g

Dietary Fiber: 1g

Sugar: 2.2g

Protein: 70.1g

Ingredient Nutritional Analysis:

Garlic

Cancer is one of the most feared diseases in the modern world. To tackle it, humans have developed many high-technology therapies, such as chemotherapy, tomotherapy, targeted therapy and antibody therapy. However, all these therapies have their own adverse side effects. Therefore, recent research has been channeled towards natural food for complementary therapy. Naturally, they have less side effects.

Garlic is one of the most powerful foods. It has been used for many centuries for both culinary and medicinal purposes. Garlic induces cancer cell death by apoptosis, autophagy and necrosis. Studies have shown how natural foods regulate cell survival or death by autophagy in cancer cells. Many ongoing researches have shown that garlic not only induces apoptosis, but also autophagy in cancerous cells.

CONCLUSION

It has been a real journey. This book has intimately discussed autophagy. With the knowledge gained from its pages, every reader has now been armed with the greatest weapon to fight against ill health or disease.

This book was adapted to suit the needs of different individuals (people facing different conditions). Autophagy helps you manage your health properly. You can only get what you invest. This applies to business, and even your body. **When you see your body as an investment**, with the dividends now being good health and long life, you would have no problems in making these adaptations (changes to achieve autophagy).

We all know the popular saying **"garbage in and garbage out"**. If you eat unhealthily, you would most likely be unhealthy. But if you eat healthy, you would likely live a healthy and fulfilled life. Best of all, eating healthy is not expensive. It simply requires you to adopt a healthy meal plan. If you properly follow the tips and steps provided in this book, in no distant time, you will reap the amazing benefits of autophagy.

This book is so rich with details that it allows you to have your cake and eat it (achieve autophagy with minimal stress). Oh yes! You will be exposed to life changing information, simplified to make execution easy.

INTERMITTENT FASTING 16/8:

Eat What You Love, Lose Weight, Increase Energy and Heal Your Body With This Lifestyle.

Includes Delicious Fat Burning Recipes

By Jaida Ellison

INTRODUCTION

First of all, fasting is not starvation. Starvation is the involuntary abstinence from eating, forced upon a person by outside forces; this happens in times of war and famine when food is scarce. Fasting, on the other hand, is voluntary, deliberate, and controlled. Food is readily available but we choose not to eat it due to spiritual, health, or other reasons.

Fasting is as old as mankind, far older than any other forms of dieting. Ancient civilizations, like the Greeks, recognized that there was something intrinsically beneficial to periodic fasting. They were often called times of healing, cleansing, purification, or detoxification. Virtually every culture and religion on earth practices some sort of ritual fasting.

Before the advent of agriculture, humans never ate three meals a day plus snacking in between. We ate only when we found food, which could be hours or days apart. Hence, from an evolutionary standpoint, eating three meals a day is not a requirement for survival. Otherwise, we would not have survived as a species.

Fast forward to the 21st century, and we have all forgotten about this ancient practice. After all, fasting is really bad for business! Food manufacturers encourage us to eat multiple meals and snacks a day. Nutritional authorities warn that skipping a single meal will have dire health consequences. Over time, these messages have been well-drilled into our heads.

Fasting has no standard duration. It may be done for a few hours to many days to months on end. Intermittent fasting is an eating pattern where we cycle between fasting and regular eating. Shorter fasts of 16-20 hours are generally done more frequently, even daily. Longer fasts, typically 24-36 hours, are done 2-3 times per week. As it happens, we all fast daily for a period of 12 hours or so between dinner and breakfast.

Fasting has been done by millions and millions of people for thousands of years. Is it unhealthy? No. In fact, numerous studies have shown that it has enormous health benefits.

This has become an extremely popular topic in the science community due to all the potential benefits for fitness and health that are being discovered.

CHAPTER ONE: Intermittent Fasting (IF)

Fasting, or periods of voluntary abstinence from food, has been practised throughout the world for ages. Intermittent fasting with the goal of improving health is relatively new. Intermittent fasting involves restricting intake of food for a set period of time and does not include any changes to the actual foods you are eating. Currently, the most common IF protocols are a daily 16 hour fast, and then fasting for a whole day, one or two days per week. Intermittent fasting could be considered a natural eating pattern that humans are built to implement, and it traces all the way back to our paleolithic hunter-gatherer ancestors. The current model of a planned program of intermittent fasting could potentially help improve many aspects of health, from body composition to longevity and aging. Although IF goes against the norms of our culture and common daily routine, the science may be pointing to a lower meal frequency and more time fasting as the optimal alternative to the normal breakfast, lunch, and dinner model. Here are two common myths that pertain to intermittent fasting.

Comparing intermittent fasting with diet fads

People experiencing intermittent fasting have proved that it does not cause starvation, tiredness, and other symptoms of daily dieting. It is because it is not the same as diet fads. It is completely different and has completely different results.

Everyone already knows dieting as a general way of losing fat. It is free of charge, simple and easy. However, the result it gives is not easy when compared to the hard work someone must go through while dieting. Sure, diets will help people lose weight, but it will not be a drastic change, and this change will probably take place after a few weeks of dieting. This is where the difference lies between diets and intermittent fasting. Following a flexible short-term fasting pattern will give an incredible result.

Not only will it reduce weight fast, but it will also show a drastic change in the body. This method affects the lifestyle of those doing the weight loss program. So, it can be a long lasting weight loss program. Another difference is that the phrase 'burn fat feed muscle' applies in intermittent fasting. Many people have proved while following this type of method that they did not lose any muscle mass.

Health benefits of intermittent fasting

- Increases Metabolism, Leading To Weight And Body Fat Loss

Unlike a daily caloric reduction diet, intermittent fasting raises the metabolism. This makes sense from a survival standpoint. If we do not eat, the body uses stored energy as fuel so that we can stay alive to find another meal. Hormones allow the body to switch energy sources from food to body fat.

Studies demonstrate this phenomenon clearly. For example, four days of continuous fasting increased the Basal Metabolic Rate by 12%. Levels of the neurotransmitter norepinephrine, which prepares the body for action, increased by 117%. Fatty acids in the bloodstream increased over 370% as the body switched from burning food to burning stored fats.

- No Loss In Muscle Mass

Unlike a constant calorie-restriction diet, intermittent fasting does not burn muscles as many have feared. In 2010, researchers looked at a group of subjects who underwent 70 days of alternate daily fasting (ate one day and fasted the next). Their muscle mass started off at 52.0 kg and ended at 51.9 kg. In other words, there was no loss of muscles but they did lose 11.4% of fat and saw major improvements in LDL cholesterol and triglyceride levels.

During fasting, the body naturally produces more human growth hormone to preserve lean muscles and bones. Muscle mass is generally preserved until body fat drops below 4%. Therefore, most people are not at risk of muscle-wasting when doing intermittent fasting.

- Reverses insulin resistance, type 2 diabetes, and fatty liver

Type 2 diabetes is a condition whereby there is simply too much sugar in the body, to the point that the cells can no longer respond to insulin and take in any more glucose from the blood (insulin resistance), resulting in high blood sugar. Also the liver becomes loaded with fat as it tries to clear out the excess glucose by converting it to and storing it as fat.

Therefore, to reverse this condition, two things have to happen:

1. Stop putting more sugar into the body.

2. Burn the remaining sugar off.

The best diet to achieve this is a low-carbohydrate, moderate-protein, and high-healthy fat diet also called the ketogenic diet. (Remember that carbohydrate raises blood sugar the most, protein to some degree, and fat the least.) That is why a low-carb diet will help reduce the burden of incoming glucose. For some people, this is already enough to reverse insulin resistance and type 2 diabetes. However, in more severe cases, diet alone is not sufficient.

What about exercise? Exercise will help burn off glucose in the skeletal muscles but not in all the tissues and organs, like the fatty liver. Clearly exercise is important, but to eliminate the excess glucose in the organs, there is the need to temporarily "starve" the cells.

Intermittent fasting can accomplish this. That is why, historically, people called fasting a cleanse or detox. It can be a very powerful tool to get rid of all the excesses. It is the fastest way to lower blood glucose and insulin levels and eventually reverse insulin resistance, type 2 diabetes, and fatty liver.

Taking insulin for type 2 diabetes does not address the root cause of the problem, which is excess sugar in the body. It is true that insulin will drive the glucose away from the blood, resulting in lower blood glucose, but where does the sugar go? The liver is just going to turn it all into fat; fat in the liver and fat in the abdomen. Patients who go on insulin often end up gaining more weight, which worsens their diabetes.

- Enhances heart health

Over time, high blood glucose from type 2 diabetes can damage the blood vessels and nerves that control the heart. The longer one has diabetes, the higher the chances that heart disease will develop. By lowering blood sugar through intermittent fasting, the risk of cardiovascular disease and stroke is also reduced.

In addition, intermittent fasting has been shown to improve blood pressure, total and LDL (bad) cholesterol, blood triglycerides, and inflammatory markers associated with many chronic diseases.

- Boosts Brain Power

Multiple studies demonstrated fasting has many neurologic benefits, including attention and focus, reaction time, immediate memory, cognition, and generation of new brain cells. Mice studies also showed that intermittent fasting reduces brain inflammation and prevents the symptoms of Alzheimer's.

- Autophagy

Autophagy is the natural process by which our body removes out cellular junk to let new cell growth happen. It destroys parts of the cell, proteins and cell membranes which are not functioning properly.

How Autophagy Works?

It is a biological process where the key players are tiny cells called lysosomes, which contain enzymes needed to digest and break down parts of the cell that no longer function properly.

That said, there is a dangerous side because lysosomes are very effective and a prolonged state of autophagy can lead to cell death; a process called autolysis. So a certain amount of autophagy is good, but too much can be damaging for our health.

Why this Cellular Junk Removal Process is so necessary?

Our body needs to regularly clean out any junk that is lying around in our cells, or else our cells become less efficient and deteriorate. When our cells are not working properly, our body becomes more susceptible to degeneration.

Autophagy makes our bodies more efficient, stops cancerous growth and metabolic dysfunction like diabetes and obesity.

How autophagy affects our cells

With it we keep our cells healthy. Our cells need cleaning from ineffective parts to avoid an imbalance between free radical damage and the antioxidants needed to prevent it. Without it, our body will experience inflammation caused by an oxidative stress. It is also necessary to keep muscle strength as you age. By removing cellular junk, your muscle stem cells continue to repair your tissues. This is the main reason detox is so important for older athletes.

CHAPTER TWO: Intermittent Fasting Guide Using the 16:8 Fasting Method

The 16:8 method of interval fasting is the most popular and simplest variant of intermittent fasting. Here you will learn everything about intermittent fasting 16/8, including instructions and important tips so you can start immediately.

Fasting has been an integral part of many world religions and cultures around the world for millennia. Nowadays, intermittent fasting is enjoying increasing popularity due to its many health benefits. There are several types of intermittent fasting. The method of intermittent fasting 16/8 is one of the most popular variations.

The 16/8 variant of intermittent fasting is a simple, convenient and sustainable way to lose weight and improve overall health enormously.

In this chapter, I'll give you an exact guide to intermittent fasting 16/8 and explain how it works and if it is right for you.

What is Intermittent Fasting 16/8?

The 16:8 method of intermittent fasting is simple and effective at the same time. Interval Fast 16/8 means limiting the consumption of food and caloric beverages to a fixed time window of eight hours a day, and dispensing with food for the remaining 16 hours. This fasting cycle can be repeated any number of times - from just once or twice a week to daily interval fasting.

With this method, your daily time window for taking meals is limited to 8 hours. The remaining 16 hours you fast and take no food. Within the 8-hour dining window, you can take 2-3 meals. This method is also known as**Leangains Protocol** and was known by fitness expert **Martin Berkhan.**

The 16/8 method of intermittent fasting is, in principle, quite simple, since your last meal of the day is dinner and you just skip breakfast the next morning. Interval fast 16/8 is a very popular form of fasting, especially if you want to lose weight fast and burn fat.

While other diets often set strict rules and waivers, 16/8 interval fasting is very easy to follow and can deliver impressive results with minimal effort. It is generally considered to be less restrictive and more flexible than many other diets and can be integrated into almost any lifestyle.

In addition to the positive effects on fat loss, 16/8 interval fasting also improves blood sugar levels and it has been proven that brain function and life expectancy are increased.

What Happens During Intermittent Fasting In The Body?

The intermittent fasting after the 16/8 variant is the trigger for a number of positive changes in your body – right down to the cellular level.

The insulin level decreases during your fasting interval, which improves insulin sensitivity. In addition, the blood sugar level is optimized and you turn yourself into a veritable fat burning engine.

A key advantage of short-term fasting is the persistent increase in human growth hormone (HGH), an important hormone involved in cell regeneration that maintains muscle mass during fasting and participates in the metabolism of body fat.

Short-term fasting also triggers important cellular repair processes in the body called autophagy. This ensures that waste and toxins are removed from the cells to keep the body healthy.

Other studies suggest that intermittent fasting is an effective defense against chronic disease and brain aging by making good changes to certain genes and molecules in your body.

Instructions For Interval Fasting 16/8

Interval fast 16/8 is easy, safe and without problems caused by needing to hold out for a long time. To start with intermittent fasting 16/8, first set an eight-hour window and limit your food intake to that amount of time.

I would recommend you to eat between 12.00 and 20.00. For many, it's the best time to eat at IF 16/8, as you'll be fasting overnight and just skip breakfast the next morning. For your first meal of the day, you will then lunch at 12.00 clock. So you do not eat and instead fast for 16 hours.

With a meal window from noon to 8pm, you can still have a well-balanced lunch and dinner and a few small afternoon snacks.

Example of a daily schedule and instructions for IF 16/8:

Your day starts at 7:00

Immediately after getting up your fat burning is highest

You skip breakfast - do not eat food - coffee is ok (no milk, no sugar)

In the morning you drink a lot of still water, coffee helps, if you feel a little hungry

At 12 o'clock you take your first meal of the day

No fast food or ready made pizza! Pay attention to a healthy meal (vegetables, salad, meat, fish, etc.)

In the afternoon you can have your second meal in the form of a small snack (a handful of nuts, hard-boiled eggs, yogurt, cereals, etc.)

At around 8:00 pm, you will have dinner and you will take your last meal of the day

After that, your 16 hour fast will start

The goal of IF is to keep your insulin levels low. Every time we eat food, insulin levels increase.

Milk in coffee, soda, sugary drinks, etc. All of this causes your insulin levels to rise and should be avoided during your 16-hour fasting phase!

When you first start interval fasting, your body is still used to having breakfast every morning. You'll probably always get hungry at the times you eat your breakfast. This is completely normal. Your body has "noticed" which food is fed at certain times.

Now that you know breakfast takes longer to appear, your body releases at the time of day at which you normally eat a breakfast that hunger hormone called ghrelin. But do not worry, that will lessen after a few days and before you know it, your body has adjusted and you will not be hungry in the morning.

I've been practicing interval fasting 16/8 in combination with a ketogenic diet for over 2 years now. And I actually do not feel hungry before 13-14, although I get up very early.

There are also people who prefer to eat between 9:00 and 17:00. At this time window you have time for a wholesome breakfast at 9:00 am, a normal lunch around noon and a light early dinner or snack around 4:00 pm before the 16 hour fasting phase begins.

Of course, you can experiment and choose the perfect time frame that best suits you and your everyday life. The important thing is that you are every day 16 hours fasting and eat no food in this time.

Regardless of when you eat your meals, it is recommended that you eat 2-3 small meals and snacks that are evenly distributed throughout the day. In this way, you can stabilize your blood sugar levels and control your hunger.

To maximize the health benefits of intermittent fasting, it is also important to keep your nutritious whole foods and sugar free drinks during your meal times. Eating fresh and nutrient-rich foods can help you improve your diet and enable the tremendous benefits of this diet with intermittent fasting.

Each meal should be combined with a good selection of healthy whole foods, such as:

- Fruit: apples, bananas, berries, oranges, peaches, pears, etc.

- Vegetables: broccoli, cauliflower, cucumbers, leafy vegetables, tomatoes,etc.

- Whole foods: quinoa, rice, oatmeal, barley, buckwheat, etc.

- Healthy fats : olive oil, avocados and coconut oil

- Protein sources: meat, poultry, fish, legumes, eggs, nuts, seeds, etc.

Non-calorific drinks such as water and unsweetened tea and coffee are allowed on interval fast 16/8. Even during fasting, these drinks can help to curb your appetite while improving hydration.

Unhealthy foods, lots of sugar and junk food can even negate the positive effects of intermittent fasting and end up doing more harm than good for your health.

Advantages Of The Intermittent Fasting 16/8 Method

The 16-8 intermittent fasting is a popular diet because it is easy to follow and flexible.

As a side benefit, you'll save even more time and money during fasting which you would otherwise spend every week cooking and preparing meals.

In terms of health, 16/8 fasting has a long list of unique benefits:

-More Fat Loss : Restricting food intake to a few hours a day not only helps reduce calories throughout the day, but studies also show that fasting boosts metabolism and increases weight loss.

-Improved glycemic control : Intermittent fasting has been found to lower insulin levels by up to 31% and blood sugar levels by 3-6%, potentially reducing the risk of diabetes.

-Better brain function : Studies show that intermittent fasting can help to form new nerve cells to promote improved brain function.

-Longer life expectancy : Although studies on humans are not yet sufficient, some animal studies have shown that intermittent fasting can extend lifespans.

Important Tips For 16-hour Fasting

Intermittent fasting is associated with many health benefits. However, it also has some disadvantages and may not be suitable for everyone.

Restricting food intake to just eight hours a day may cause some people to eat more than usual during mealtimes to make up for the hours of fasting. This can lead to weight gain, digestive problems and the establishment of unhealthy eating habits.

Intermittent fasting 16/8 can also cause short-term side effects such as hunger, depression, and fatigue. However, these "side effects" are shortlived and can be overcome after a few days, when you get into a routine and get used to the interval fasting.

In addition, some scientific evidence suggests that intermittent fasting may affect men and women differently, with animal testing demonstrating that it may affect fertility in women.

However, it has to be said that more human studies are needed to reliably assess the impact of intermittent fasting on reproductive health in women.

In any case, you should start gradually and consider consulting your doctor if you have any concerns or have negative symptoms.

Is intermittent fasting 16/8 suitable for me?

Intermittent fasting with the 16/8 method can be a sustainable, safe and easy way to improve your health.

Especially when short-term fasting is combined with an off-balance diet, a ketogenic nutritional plan and a healthy lifestyle.

Intervall fasting is not a diet! Rather, it is a way of eating nutrionally but should not be considered a substitute for a balanced and wholesome diet.

Although intermittent fasting is generally considered safe for most healthy adults, you should talk to your doctor before you start, especially if you have any health problems, prescriptions, diabetes, low blood pressure, or an earlier eating disorder.

Intermittent fasting is also not recommended for all women, especially when trying to get pregnant or for women who are pregnant or nursing.

If you are concerned about whether IF 16/8 is for you, or if you experience unwanted side effects while fasting, be sure to visit your family doctor.

Conclusion

During IF 16/8 you limit your food intake to an 8-hour window and for the remaining 16 hours you fast. It is very effective because it allows the body to reach the highest level of fat burning that occurs about 8-12 hours after eating a meal. In addition, intermittent fasting 16/8 supports weight loss, improves blood sugar levels, brain function and increases overall life expectancy.

Eat above all healthy foods during your 8-hour window and drink noncaloric beverages such as water or unsweetened tea and coffee (excluding milk and sugar).

If you have any health problems, it is always a good idea to talk to your doctor first before you start intermittent fasting.

Important FAQ'S: Intermittent Fasting 16:8

1. Where does the 16:8 interval fasting come from?

Phases of fasting are nothing new to our body. In ancient times, it was normal for our ancestors to have their stomachs empty for hours or days in times of scarcity. Once food was available, the reserves were replenished extensively.

As a rule, the body easily survives small starvation periods by storing energy reserves in various organs and tissues. If necessary, it can then fall back on this energy.

2.What must be taken care of during the 16:8 interval fasting?

It is important not to eat more in the phases of food intake than is usually consumed per meal. You should also pay attention to what you eat instead of indulging indiscriminately during the eight hours.

In addition, it is advisable to take only two meals and in between a break of 4 - 5 hours. If you take carbohydrates in between, no matter if they are biscuits, bread, dairy products or even fruit juices, then the body converts them into sugar. It goes directly into the blood. As a result the blood sugar level rises, insulin is released and the body stops fat loss. In addition, it may increasingly lead to food cravings.

3.No success in the 16:8 Interval fast: Why do not I take off weight with this?

If you do not lose weight despite the fasting phases, it may be because you just eat too much in the food phases. If you eat more than your body consumes, you lose the benefits of fasting.

Another reason may be the choice of food. Those who only eat unhealthy, high-calorie and sugary foods during the 8 hours can not hope for weight loss success. Only in connection with a healthy diet, the 16:8 fasting can lead to weight loss.

4.How much can you lose in 16:8 interval fasting?

Each body responds differently to a diet, and how much one ultimately decreases depends on different things. On the one hand, how overweight you were at the beginning of the fasting can make a difference, because the more body fat you have, the more the body can of course also break down.

On the other hand, weight loss depends on how you feed yourself and how much exercise you do during your time, for example.

5.Which drinks and food are particularly suitable for the 16:8 interval fasting?

Especially if you want to reduce your weight, the following foods and drinks are suitable:

- A lot of fresh fruits and vegetables
- Nuts and dried fruit as a snack, instead of biscuits and chips
- Protein and fiber-rich foods
- Silent waters
- Unsweetened teas
- Black, unsweetened coffee
- Superfoods such as chia seeds

6.Breakfast or dinner: which meal should be suspended?

The 16:8 interval fast is relatively well integrated into everyday life, no matter if you are an early riser or a night person. Lent extends over the night and part of the morning and evening.

If you are reluctant to have breakfast, the method will not be a problem and you can start with lunch as your first meal and then have time for a late dinner.

If you do not want to miss your breakfast, you can skip dinner and have your last meal in the afternoon.

Another option is to have breakfast late and have dinner early, for example, between 11:00 and 19:00.

7.In which pre-existing conditions one should not fast according to the 16:8 method?

Do not use the IF 16:8 for the following pre-existing conditions:

- cardiovascular disorders
- chronic diseases
- metabolic diseases

- low blood pressure Besides,

not:

- during pregnancy and lactation with
- eating disorders or underweight

8.How do you do it in a safe way?

To follow the 16:8 diet safely, you must drink enough while you are not eating. Coffee or unsweetened green tea can be helpful (or pre-workout) the morning before exercise, as long as you do not use sweeteners or cream.

Consumption of a BCAA supplement is believed to prevent fasting muscle loss just prior to exercise. In the 8-hour meal period, it is essential to provide high-quality meals with all the necessary macronutrients, vitamins and minerals for the day. Continue to drink enough and add enough protein to prevent loss of muscle mass. It can be hard to get enough calories in this short time, which can lead to weakness and dizziness.

In addition, you should be careful not to eat too much in your 8 hours just because there are 16 hours of fasting ahead of you. Intermittent fasting is designed to keep the body in a deficit for the day as a whole, so you should not over-feed high-calorie foods.

9.When is the best time to play sports?

Basically, the best time to do sports is the end of the Lenten window.

This way you can provide your body with all the valuable and important nutrients right in your food phase.

However, a sports unit should not be taken right after the last meal, as it may make you hungry in your next fasting phase.

CHAPTER THREE: Other Types of Intermittent Fasting

1. 24-HOUR FASTING

You don't have to fast for days or weeks to reap the benefits of this amazing weight loss and cleansing practice. Water and lemon juice fasting can do wonders for our digestion system and our entire body.

One easy way to get you started is trying the 24 hour fast! This is a great way to give fasting a try. It is also very beneficial to your overall health. Let's discuss this in more detail.

Fasting is done in two basic ways 1) Water Fasting and 2) Juice Fasting. Water fasting is recommended for experienced fasters only. Juice fasting is much more user-friendly and is very effective. People can fast anywhere from 1-30 days, although some people do go for longer. For most people, a 1-3 day fast is the best way to go and this will benefit you immensely.

Here Are The Guidelines

- **Hours of Fast** - I think the easiest is dinner to dinner so about 6PM6PM. Why? Well, you are asleep part of the time, therefore your body is resting and you are not thinking about food. It seems to flow well with most peoples' schedules. Anytime is okay though, depending upon your schedule.
- **Before the Fast** - Eat lightly several hours before the fasting period. Don't stuff yourself with solid and heavy food. Eat healthy and light foods only.

- **Drink Juice -** Drink lots of juice. I favor non-pasteurized green juice and carrot/beet, but any vegetable combo is great. If it's difficult to find non-pasteurized juice at least buy organic/natural non-filtered juice. Lemon Juice with water (made from squeezing organic lemons) is another great way to help the body cleanse. And again some people use cranberry juice, but it needs to be pure juice, no sugar or concentrate. Any juice is good, but organic is best, natural only, and it should be only pure juice and water, with no other ingredients. • **Drink Cleansing Tea** - Herbal & Green Teas help the process of cleansing your body. There are several fasting and detox teas, my favorites are made by Yogi Tea and Traditional Medicinals, or you can make your own. Cleansing teas and herbs are available at most natural food stores or online. Herbs are an essential way to help the fasting and cleanse process. Drink a few cups during your fast.
- **Drink Water -** Water will cleanse and filter out toxins. Drink lots of filtered water, which of course includes tea and juice. Pure filtered water is essential for your cleanse and overall health.
- **Eliminate Toxins -** Urinate and have bowel movements as much as you can. You will urinate frequently as you are drinking liquids. Tea and Raw juice, and in particular vegetable juices, will help you eliminate solid waste and cleanse your colon.

2. THE WARRIOR DIET

If you are one of those people who hate eating breakfast and find it much more convenient and enjoyable to eat one large meal rather than several small meals a day then you will not find the Warrior diet interesting but very enjoyable. The diet is based on the habits of ancient warriors who, in preparing for battle, ate little during the day but enjoyed a huge meal at night when they were less likely to be attacked and therefore could rest and enjoy their food.

Rather than a diet, it is a more an overall fitness program that combines diet, exercise and sound nutrition in a kind of feast or famine arrangement. The idea behind the diet is that during the day when you should be most active, you should eat very little. Eating a very small amount of food with no or limited protein stresses the body, making you burn calories faster, and adds to mental alertness. While this is only a theory many of you know from your own experience how you often feel sleepy shortly after eating, so the theory does make a lot of sense. By eating near to nothing your body and your mind are more alert because they aren't sated.

How Does It Work and Why Is It Beneficial?

This diet was devised by Ori Holmekler who suggests that it is not for bodybuilding, but instead for a way to develop a lean muscular body while at the same time keeping your size and weight down, in essence giving you a Bruce Lee look.

This diet works because of how your nervous system is set up to handle the digestion of food and funnelling of available energy. During the 20 hours that you are under eating, the Sympathetic Nervous System (SNS) is responsible for your ability to deal with stress, physical activity and periods of intense concentration. Basically anytime you need energy or cohesive body function it is the responsibility of the SNS to provide you with it. Whenever you eat, the SNS gets turned off as the parasympathetic nervous system (PNS) gets turned on, which is responsible for the digestion of food. This is why after having a big lunch it is common to have energy crashes and feel like taking a nap as opposed to carrying on with the day. Taking a nap anytime you eat a meal or a snack does sound nice, but who in this day and age has the time for that?

The overeating phase of the Warrior Diet will typically be during 4 hours of the evening. The PNS will be maximized during this time and will aid in resting, digestion and detoxification, among other things. All food groups will need to be consumed during this period of time; however, it does not mean that you should binge on junk food and sugary snacks. Usually, this will not be a problem because a person on this diet will crave the foods that the body actually needs as opposed to the foods that one might crave if they wanted to indulge their taste buds only. Of course, during the first few weeks or even months, there will be a transition period where you will need to condition yourself to lose the cravings for your old eating habits. This can be particularly difficult if you have a strong reliance on sugary foods and drinks. It has been said that a person's desire for food is the hardest to suppress, so this diet really does put this statement to the test.

3. ONE MEAL A DAY (OMAD)

OMAD stands for One Meal a Day; the idea is to fast for 23 hours straight and then consume one large meal in a 60-minute window.

Normally this involves waiting until dinner to break your OMAD fast, but ultimately it could be any meal with a 23:1 fast (it can technically be a 22:2 plan as well if you eat your one meal's worth of food slowly). People typically do OMAD to improve their health, lose weight, or both.

Because OMAD is a more advanced way to intermittent fast, it is a chance to get in on all the research-backed benefits like:

1. Increased human growth hormone (HGH) levels, which allows us toactually build muscle and burn fat

2. Lowered inflammation levels

3. Decreased disease risks

4. Increased autophagy pathways (cellular recycling and repair)

Another key benefit of fasting techniques like OMAD is that they enhance nutritional ketosis, which has its own anti-inflammatory, fat-burning, and autophagy benefits. Because OMAD is a longer fast, it tends to maximize these benefits. Longer fasting windows give the body longer periods of time to enhance all the benefits of fasting; breaking the fast earlier slows those mechanisms.

4. ALTERNATE DAY FASTING

This type of diet is based upon "calorie shifting" principles. Calorie shifting is a scientifically proven method of losing weight by eating more calories one day and fewer the next. The diets we will examine here follow these principles, but do so in different ways. The biggest advantage of eating this way is the effect it has on your metabolism. By making your body think it is not dieting, your metabolism will continue running high and your weight loss will happen faster and for longer periods.

Below Are Descriptions Of The Most Popular Alternative Day Fasting Diets:

- **QOD Diet**

The QOD Diet is a diet program based on a book that is all about on days and off days. On your "On Days" you are allowed to eat fairly regularly, but you must watch your sodium and potassium intake. On your "Off Days," you are relegated to eat only 500 calories and only 200 of them are allowed to come from protein. Again you are asked to limit sodium and potassium.

On top of that, you are asked to take supplements and protein powders to help regulate what you ingest. This will help facilitate faster weight loss according to the creators of this alternate day diet plan.

- **Up Day Down Day Diet**

This diet takes the QOD Diet a little farther because it does not require using so many supplements and potions to help with weight loss. It starts with the induction phase where you are on "Up Days and Down Days" (sounds familiar right?). During induction, you will be restricted to 500 calories and you are not as constrained by sodium and potassium. This makes the diet a little easier than the QOD. On down days you are allowed to eat regularly as long as you don't "purposely overeat"

That last statement is a little more ambiguous and tough when you are starving yourself the day before.

After the induction phase, you go to the maintenance phase where your down days are eating 50% of your normal eating routine.

- **The Every Other Day Diet (EODD)**

The EODD goes even further towards the ultimate alternate day diet. The EODD has different phases like the Up Day Down Day Diet, but they work the same in each phase. The reason this diet is more refined is that it incorporates the SNAPP Eating Plan which tells you exactly what to eat. So on "Burn" days, you eat exactly what the SNAPP Plan tells you.

On "Feed" days you can eat pizza, hamburgers etc. as long as it is during the times outlined in SNAPP. The rest of the meals you eat what's told in the plan.

5. FASTING MIMICKING DIET

Fast mimicking is a type of modified fasting. Instead of abstaining from food completely like a traditional fast, you still consume small amounts of food in a way that produces the therapeutic benefits of fasting.

A fast mimicking diet typically lasts about five days and follows a healthy protocol low in carbs, protein, and calories and high in fat. Calories are kept at around 40% of normal intake. This allows the body to stay nourished with nutrients and electrolytes will give you less stress than normal fasting but while still receiving the same benefits.

Long-term calorie restriction and long-term fasting can harmful, but fast mimicking is safer and more effective. Let's look at how much it differs from traditional fasting.

According to the advice of the World Health Organisation, consuming these five a day portions will assist any average person in reducing their risks of suffering heart disease, a stroke or a variety of cancers. The diet that includes these portions will also likely reduce the problems of diabetes and obesity, by helping to reduce artificial sugars in the diet and reducing our propensity in Western cultures to eat too much, which is what has led to the obesity epidemic all around us.

You eat 500-1000 calories a day for 2-5 days and on day 6 you return to a normal way of eating. It can be used for weight loss, fighting disease, and promoting longevity. Here's how it works:

- You eat about 500-1000 calories every day.
- Your daily macros are low protein, moderate carb, moderate fat. You
- eat things like a nutbar, a bowl of soup, and some crackers with a few olives or something.

- Day One you eat about 1000 calories – 10% protein, 55% fat, and 35% carbs.
- Day 2-5 you eat about 500-700 calories – 10% protein, 45% fat, 45% carbs.
- Day 6 you transition back to a normal caloric intake with complex carbs, vegetables, and minimal meat, fish, and cheese.

6. PROTEIN SPARING MODIFIED FASTING

The idea of a PSMF is to reduce calories to the lowest possible threshold while still eating enough protein to preserve lean tissue mass and enough micronutrients to avoid deficiency. This is basically a kind of starvation, so you get the same metabolic benefits that you do with a "real" fast (which is also basically a kind of starvation), but the additional protein and nutrients make the whole project a little less risky and minimize muscle loss and potential nutrient deficiencies.

Practically, a PSMF involves:

Very few calories (typically under 1,000 per day – remember that the point is to induce a starvation response), with the vast majority coming from lean protein. Fat and carbs are minimized as much as possible.

A few non-starchy vegetables.

Supplemental vitamins, minerals, and salts to make up the inevitable nutrient and electrolyte deficiencies.

On a PSMF, the majority of calories entering your mouth are from protein, but the majority of calories you burn for energy come from fat; patients on a PSMF do go into ketosis. That's because you can't "burn" protein for energy the way you burn fat or carbs. The protein is just there to replenish muscle mass and prevent lean tissue loss – it's used as building blocks, not as fuel. Instead of burning that protein for fuel, you'll be burning your own body fat reserves so you essentially are "eating" fat – your own fat.

A PSMF consists of two phases. The first "intensive" phase lasts 4-6 months and involves severely limiting calories.

The second "refeeding" phase lasts 6-8 weeks, during which calories are gradually increased back to a more regular level.

7. FAT FASTING

A fat fast is a high-fat, low-calorie diet that typically lasts 2–5 days.

During this time it's recommended to eat 1,000–1,200 calories per day, 80–90% of which should come from fat.

Though not technically a fast, this approach mimics the biological effects of abstaining from food by putting your body into the biological state of ketosis.

In ketosis your body uses fat, rather than carbs, as its main energy source. During this process, your liver breaks down fatty acids into molecules called ketones, which can be used to fuel your body.

Ketosis occurs during times when glucose, your body's main source of energy, isn't available, such as during periods of starvation or when your carb intake is very low.

The time it takes to achieve ketosis can vary considerably, but if you're following a ketogenic diet you can typically expect to reach this state between days 2 and 6.

Fat fasting is designed to get you into ketosis quickly or to boost ketone levels if you have already achieved ketosis by restricting both your calorie and carb intake.

It's usually used by people on a ketogenic diet who want to break through an ongoing weight loss plateau or by those wanting to get back into ketosis after a cheat day, on which the rules of a low-carb diet are relaxed and you eat foods that are high in carbs.

A fat fast is very low in calories and high in fat. It's designed to create a calorie deficit, which is needed for weight loss, while quickly depleting your body's carb stores so you move into ketosis and burn more fat.

Thus if you adhere to this protocol strictly for 2–5 days, you may enter ketosis and begin burning fat as your primary source of fuel, particularly if you're already on a very-low-carb diet.

Nonetheless, a fat fast only last a few days, so large shifts on the scale can't be explained by fat loss alone.

The loss of your body's carb stores also leads to a loss of water, which is stored alongside glycogen, the stored form of glucose. This gives the illusion of fat loss.

8. BONE BROTH FASTING

A bone broth fast means you consume bone broth several times per day but not much other solid food. Fasts are not for everyone, and sometimes certain kinds can pose risks since they involve consuming little nutrients due to greatly reducing calorie intake. However, if you make a good candidate, consuming bone broth is ideal for a fast because it's chock-full of important macronutrients and micronutrients, including amino acids (which form proteins) like glycine, arginine and proline; vitamins and minerals; collagen; electrolytes; and even antioxidants like glucosamine.

Most people do best fasting for a period between three to four days, during this time consuming several quarts of bone broth daily and eliminating many problematic foods. One of the things that makes a bone broth fast stand apart from other types of fasts is that it's an ideal way to obtain more collagen, which is a type of protein needed to create healthy tissue found throughout the body. Collagen is found inside the lining of the digestive tract, within bones in bone marrow, in skin, and in the tissues that form joints, tendons, ligaments and cartilage.

Within collagen are other special nutrients, including amino acids like proline and glycine, plus gelatin which all have widespread benefits.

How To Start A Bone Broth Fast

Typically the fast lasts anywhere between 24 hours and 3 days, but we recommend starting small if you're new to fasting or consuming a diet high in processed food.

Most bone broth fasts consist of consuming between 3 to 4 quarts of bone broth per day while avoiding solid food and intense exercise. Fasting allows your body to burn fat, boost your metabolism, and heal conditions such as leaky gut due to its ability to restore good bacteria in the digestive tract. When you add in the numerous benefits of bone broth protein, the electrolyte and amino acid content hydrates, these come togeter to detox and heal your body.

Most fasting is done without solid food. However, if you are new to fasting or are feeling light-headed, it's okay to include one small meal of grass-fed meat and vegetables for every 24 hours of fasting.

9. DRY FASTING

Dry fasting is a type of fast that doesn't allow any water intake. The lack of water may help accelerate some of the protective effects you get on a regular water fast, like reduced inflammation and metabolic health.

However, it's a more advanced fasting method that only people who have previous experience with normal fasts should attempt.

Dry fasting has been perfected and practiced by many cultures and religions throughout history:

- Judaism (during Yom Kippur)
- Christianity (during Lent and Advent)
- Mormonism (one Sunday of each month)
- Buddhism (to aid meditation)
- Jainism (to reach transcendence)
- Islam (during Ramadan)

The Islamic, Mormon, and Jewish fasts are the only ones that prohibit water, so they're true dry fasts.

There Are Two Popular Types Of Dry Fasting Methods.

Hard and soft dry fasting is very popular. With the hard dry fast, the faster does not even allow water to touch their body. None!

When dry fasting the pores of the skin absorb water from contact with the environment.

This is one of the reasons many dry fasting experts believe it is best to practice in the outdoors, in the mountains as opposed to in cities.

This much cleaner environment is preferred as the skin absorbs water through the moisture in the air. Sleeping outside and near running water in this environment is ideal for longer dry fasting.

As you can imagine, the soft dry fast allows the participant to drink water during the fast. The presence of water lessens the beneficial and the uncomfortable effects of dry fasting but allows the faster to fast for longer periods of time. This is preferred for beginners.

10. JUICE FASTING

Juice fasting is a great way to get off the dieting rollercoaster and see real results quickly. Safe and effective when carried out correctly, juice fasting benefits your entire being.

Your physical wellbeing increases as the body is rid of toxins and excess fat.

Your mind benefits because fasting creates a stillness that brings mental clarity and helps you to develop will power and to better control your senses.

As you lose weight and feel much better about yourself, self-esteem improves and sets you on the road to what could be a life-changing experience, connecting you to your spirit and helping you to achieve balance in your life.

General Juicing Rules:

- Drink freshly prepared juice and do not store the juice for over 24 hours. If you can't drink it immediately, put it into a glass jar (filled to the top) and put a lid on it to prevent oxidation. Juice rapidly loses therapeutic and nutritional value during storage.
- Raw fruits and vegetables are not always compatible when eaten together. Apples are the exception. You can also mix pears with Jicama.
- Melons should be juiced by themselves. Making the entire meal melon is an option.
- Avoid using pre-bottled or sweetened juices. All the live enzymes are inactivated when they are pasteurized.
- Juices don't stimulate acids to be released from the stomach, but orange and tomato juice are high in acids and you may want to mix these juices with other less acidic ones.
- Don't add more than 25% green juice to your vegetable juices. (Unless you have a barf bucket handy!)
- Juicing Greens--you might want to do this in between harder vegetables, as the juice sludges at the bottom and doesn't pour out easily if you juice them first.
- Dilute all fruit juice with water (one part juice to 2-4 parts water) and drink throughout the day. We've found that 2 cups fruit juice blended with ½ tray of ice cubes comes up to 4 cups--the perfect dilution and it's frothy cold.

- Vegetable juices need not be diluted.

11.TIME-RESTRICTED FEEDING

If you know anyone that has said they are doing intermittent fasting, odds are it is in the form of time-restricted feeding. This is a type of intermittent fasting that is used daily and it involves only consuming calories during a small portion of the day and fasting for the remainder.

Daily fasting intervals in time-restricted feeding may range from 12-20 hours, with the most common method being 16/8 (fasting for 16 hours, consuming calories for 8). For this protocol, the time of day is not important as long as you are fasting for a consecutive period of time and only eating in your allowed time period.

For example, on a 16/8 time-restricted feeding program one person may eat their first meal at 7AM and last meal at 3PM (fast from 3PM-7AM), while another person may eat their first meal at 1PM and last meal at 9PM (fast from 9PM-1PM).

This protocol is meant to be performed every day over long periods of time and is very flexible as long as you are staying within the fasting/eating window(s).

Time-restricted feeding is one of the easiest to follow methods of intermittent fasting. Using this along with your daily work and sleep schedule may help achieve optimal metabolic function. Time-restricted feeding is a great program to follow for weight loss and body composition improvements, as well as some other overall health benefits. The few human trials that were conducted noted significant reductions in weight, reductions in fasting blood glucose, and improvements in cholesterol with no changes in perceived tension, depression, anger, fatigue, or confusion. Some other preliminary results from animal studies showed time-restricted feeding to protect against obesity, high insulin levels, fatty liver disease, and inflammation.

The easy application and promising results of time-restricted feeding could possibly make it an excellent option for weight loss and chronic disease prevention/management. When implementing this protocol it may be good to begin with a lower fasting-to-eating ratio like 12/12 hours and eventually work your way up to 16/8 hours.

CHAPTER FOUR

Commonly asked questions about intermittent fasting and supplements

What is the most important supplement that I should be taking?

At bare minimum, everyone should be taking a multivitamin of some sort because of nutrient deficient soil.

I prefer organic, whole food vitamin sources such as powdered greens.

-What Supplements Should I Be Taking?

A multivitamin, an omega 3 source, a probiotic, and Vitamin D. As I said before, I prefer whole food sources over artificial multivitamins. So I would use a greens source as my multivitamin. I use a high-quality fish oil or krill oil for my omega 3 source. An alternative for vegans would be flaxseed oil or hemp oil. As for probiotics, the best source is naturally fermented foods such as miso soup, kimchi, natto, kefir, and sauerkraut. As for supplementation, get one that has more than 10 billion active probiotic strains per serving. Vitamin D supplementation is very important for people who don't get at least one hour of sunlight exposure per day. For instance, if you live in the northeast US, you will definitely need it. People with darker complexions will need more sun exposure than light-skinned folks because UV-B rays do not penetrate the skin as far. Therefore, less sunlight is converted to Vitamin D. The latest studies are saying that almost everyone is deficient in Vitamin D.

-What Is The Best Type Of Protein Powder To Buy?

It depends on what you are using it for. Whey is the best all-purpose protein. It absorbs fast, is cheap, and is best taken after a workout. Casein protein is best taken before bed because it is slowly absorbed. I would stick to a protein powder that is made from grass-fed cow's milk for higher quality.

-When Should I Take My Protein Supplement: Before Or After A Workout?

If you can afford it, both. The influx of branch chained amino acids taken before will give you a better performance throughout your workout. If you are trying to save money, the optimal time to take a protein supplement is within 30 minutes of completing your workout for recovery.

- I Have Tried All Diets And They Have Failed. What's The Easiest Way To See Results Without Dieting?

Intermittent fasting may work for you. Research shows that the 18th hour is the "golden hour". This is when you see the most results for the least amount of time. There are different theories on intermittent fasting. Some say the fast starts after your last meal and others say that it starts 2 or 3 hours after your last meal due to digestion. You do not want to fast over 24 hours straight. This is where negative effects on metabolism are seen and honestly, anything over 24 hours is miserable and uncomfortable.

-What am I allowed to eat during intermittent fasting?

Intermittent fasting is about not eating for a certain amount of time. There are no restrictions during the meal phase. That means all foods are allowed. There are no permanent prohibitions! And the amount or the number of calories is not limited in intermittent fasting. Even pure junk food consumers benefit from the daily meal breaks.

-Are medications and dietary supplements allowed for interval fasting?

Medication and nutritional supplements can be taken as usual during jntermittent fasting. Most supplements can even be taken during the fasting phase because they do not disturb the fasting process. The use of medication should not be changed on your own anyway, but only in consultation with a doctor.

Since intermittent fasting may decrease high blood pressure levels and improve insulin sensitivity of the cells, people who take medication for blood pressure or blood sugar should fast intermittently under close medical supervision. Here, if necessary, an adjustment of the drug dose is needed.

- Can I drink alcohol during intermittent fasting?

Alcohol provides calories and is therefore not allowed during fasting. In the dining window, however, you can also take alcoholic drinks. A general prohibition of alcohol does not exist in intermittent fasting.

-When is the best time for sports?

In principle, you can do sports while intermittent fasting at any time, both in the fasting and in the food phase. There are no concrete rules here. If you really want to burn fat, you should train on an empty stomach, because it promotes fat metabolism and afterburning.

-How long should I fast during intermittent fasting?

Intermittent fasting can be flexibly designed. You can fast every day for 14, 16, 18, 20 hours or more. In the classic variant, the IF 16/8, 16-hour fasting phases alternate with 8-hour meal windows.

How long your meal break should ideally be during intermittent fasting is not the same for all people. Again, there are differences that are partly due to your personal neurotransmitter dominance.

It’s advisable you to start with the classic variant, ie IF 16/8, and stay for four weeks. This is the best way to find out if fasting 16 hours a day is too much or too little for you.

-Will I lose weight by intermittent fasting ?

How much you take off through interval fasting depends on various factors. Your current weight, how much overweight you are is just as important as the length of the meal break and of course, what you take during the meal phase to you.

There are numerous case reports of people who already lose weight with the IF 16/8 method without having to restrict their eating habits or count calories. Then again, there are people who have to fast for at least 18 or 20 hours without food and / or pay attention to their diet.

However, the fact is that intermittent fasting is definitely better for losing weight than traditional diets. That's because insulin levels are low for a long time due to interval fasting. This in turn is a prerequisite for the body to burn stored fat stores to energy and to keep the basal metabolic rate stable. So you lose fat faster than muscle during interval fasting, and you do not have to worry about the notorious yo-yo effect that calorie reduction diets trigger.

-How long can you interval fast?

With intermittent fasting, you do not have to do without anything permanently. There are no prohibitions. Favorite foods are still allowed. This and the flexible design of the meal breaks make intermittent fasting so incredibly attractive for long-term use.

Intermittent fasting is not a time-limited diet nor a temporary fad. This is the "original lifestyle" of man, according to his biological design and in accordance with the hormonal and neurobiological rhythms of the body standing.

Intermittent fasting is optimally suited as a permanent nutritional model in contrast to most diets. Short-term fasting can last your life - and with a clear conscience!

-Are exceptions allowed for intermittent fasting?

It may happen that invitations, parties or other occasions thwart your plans and you do not manage to keep the usual meal break. Of course this is not a broken leg. It's recommended simply making an exception and consciously enjoying it, rather than being a social outsider with astonished looks and tough discussions.

Nor is it a tragedy when 16 hours become only 14 or 12 hours. Maybe you just do not want to miss the breakfast with your loved ones at the weekend. All this is basically no problem. Practicing IF 16/8 5 or 6 days a week brings positive effects.

However, its recommened that you stay consistent for the first time of the changeover until you have become accustomed to the meal breaks. Otherwise there is a danger that you will not find the IF-rhythm after the exception.

-Can I continue the Intermittent fasting even when I am ill?

If you are ill because you have caught a cold or a flu, its better to listen to your feelings. If you are hungry, eat something, but do not force yourself to do anything. Often, when you're sick, you do not have an appetite anyway. In our eyes, this is a clear sign that the body does not need food, but puts all its forces into self-healing.

-Do I take enough nutrients with interval fasting?

Because you eat less often through interval fasting, some people are afraid that they will not get enough nutrients. However, intermittent fasting has a very positive effect on the gut. The long phases without food improve the intestinal flora and absorbed nutrients can be utilized much better again. There are no more effective measures than daily meal breaks to improve the nutritional supply!

-How often do you eat during the mealtime interval?

Basically, there is no rule for how often you should eat during interval fasting within your food window. So everyone can handle it the way they want.

People who eat small portions probably still need three meals on the 16/8 interval fasting method, which allows them to eat eight hours a day. Others, however, cope well with two large meals or a snack and a lavish main meal.

Regardless of how you decide to work it, from a physiological point of view you should not constantly snack during the food phase with intermittent fasting, but allow at least three to four hours pass between meals.

Two common myths that pertain to intermittent fasting

Myth 1 - You Must Eat 3 Meals Per Day: This "rule" that is common in Western society was not developed based on evidence for improved health, but was adopted as the common pattern for settlers and eventually became the norm. Not only is there a lack of scientific rationale in the 3 meal-a-day model, but recent studies may be showing less meals and more fasting to be optimal for human health. One study showed that one meal a day with the same amount of daily calories is better for weight loss and body composition than 3 meals per day. This finding is a basic concept that is extrapolated into intermittent fasting and those choosing to do IF may find it best to only eat 1-2 meals per day.

Myth 2 - You Need Breakfast, It's The Most Important Meal of The Day: Many false claims about the absolute need for a daily breakfast have been made. The most common claims being "breakfast increases your metabolism" and "breakfast decreases food intake later in the day". These claims have been refuted and studied over a 16 week period, with results showing that skipping breakfast did not decrease metabolism and it did not increase food intake at lunch and dinner. It is still possible to do intermittent fasting protocols while still eating breakfast, but some people find it easier to eat a late breakfast or skip it altogether and this common myth should not get in the way.

Intermittent fasting – How to do it healthily and safely

Intermittent fasting can improve health, reduce the risk of serious illness, and promote longevity. Perhaps you're intrigued and would like to give it a go but aren't sure how to start. Or maybe you have tried it once or twice and found it too challenging. Here, I will give you strategies and guidelines to practice intermittent fasting safely and successfully. Please read the contraindications at the end of this chapter before doing a fast.

Intermittent fasting can be practised in the easiest way i.e 16:8 daily, meaning 16 hrs not eating and 8 hours eating. This can be done for a few months before starting another IF. A person may decide to eat 7am to 10pm (i.e 15 hours of eating and 9 hours not eating) and later move to 10 hours eating and 14 hours not eating and so on.

Follow the below guideline to effectively practice IF:

- Pick a day that isn't too hectic or demanding because you may experience some detox reactions. Make sure you have the option to relax if you need to. You will get more out of the experience if you make time to turn inward, still the mind, meditate, contemplate, and listen to your inner guidance.
- Enlist support from people close to you before you start. It's great to fast with your partner so you can both motivate each other and share experiences.
- Eat lightly the evening before by choosing a large salad or steamed vegetables with some lean protein. There is no point gorging the night before because it will make you feel even hungrier whilst you fast. It's best to avoid alcohol as well.
- Don't fight feeling hungry because you most probably will. Just be with the sensation without judgment, rather than resisting it (but read guideline 10 below).
- Engage in light exercise such as walking, stretching, and gentle yoga. This is not the day to do an intense gym workout or anything too vigorous.

- Add some breathing exercises such as yogic pranayama. A few minutes of practice offers amazing benefits from detoxification to boosting energy.
- Expect some detox symptoms such as headaches, feeling groggy, or short periods of feeling jittery. These are made worse if you usually have lots of caffeine and sugar in your diet. Avoid taking over-thecounter medication to reduce these side effects. Instead rest, go for a walk, and practice breathing exercises.

- Listen to your body's wisdom and if you feel unwell or it gets too much then have some food. Your body knows best.
- Break the fast gently the following morning. Have water or herb tea and a piece of fruit when you get up, then 30min later have your usual breakfast. Eat as usual for the rest of the day (you probably won't feel the need to overeat).
- During the fasting time, its much recommended to drink pure water or mix 1.5 litre pure water with a cup of black coffee or tea (no sugar, ofcourse).

Enjoy the changes in how you feel during and after the fast. Notice changes in your energy, emotions, and mental state. You may notice food is far more enjoyable on the day after the fast because your senses are heightened.

Recognise that it can take a few attempts to get used to this practice. After a few weeks your body will get used to it and the benefits you feel will increase as the discomfort simultaneously decreases.

Contra-Indications:

Avoid intermittent fasting if you are pregnant, diabetic, suffering from a serious illness, or taking any prescribed medications. If in doubt it is best to consult with your health care provider.

Potential risk of intermittent fasting

The most common risk from intermittent fasting is dehydration. If you are consuming less then your body is taking on less water, it is very important you don't forget to drink on the days you do not eat. Water is essential and black coffee is often used if you get bored with plain water. With no food going in the stomach you are at risk of heartburn from stomach acid and long-term ulcers that can occur if stomach acid builds up against the stomach walls. The mental side of fasting also has to be considered. If you fast 2 days a week, don't over indulge on the other 5, keep to normal meals or it could lead someone to psychological disorders such as bulimia. You also need to be sure you are eating the right nutrients and minerals.

Continue to eat fruit and vegetables. If you don't eat for 2 days, make sure the other 5 you are eating enough fruit and vegetables and not just binging or eating convenience foods.

Proven tips to reduce hunger while doing intermittent fasting

1. Balance Your Macronutrients (Protein, Carbs, and Fats)

Most people fail on intermittent fasting because they go very low carb and keep entering a state of ketosis which can be very detrimental for short-term bursts of high-intensity activity.

Carbohydrates: Minimum 0,6g per pound of body mass to stay out of ketosis.

Some individuals will also find higher carbohydrate intakes help them feel fuller.

It's better to keep fat between 25-30% of total calorie intake.

2. Don't Mistake Hunger for Dehydration

Hunger signals are often misleading – usually, we just need water.

To get an adequate amount of water carry a refillable bottle with you and aim for a gallon a day.

3. Tea and Coffee work wonders

Drinking coffee and tea is a great way to help curb your hunger while fasting. Before getting into the "HOW", first let's clarify what kinds of coffee and tea can be consumed without breaking a fast. When looking at coffee, any kind of BLACK coffee will not break your fast!

Black Coffee = No Creamers, Milk, or Sugar!

If you really don't like black coffee and need some sweetness in it, you can add any 0 CALORIE sweetener in small amounts, such as Stevia. When it comes to tea, the same rules apply; your tea must be BLACK in order for you to stay fasted!

It is also important to note that any HERBAL TEAS which include FRUIT are a NO GO while fasting! Fruit contains glucose which will definitely break your fast! Any black or green teas are good to go, also any spice based teas (ex. ginger) are safe as well.

How does coffee and tea curb your hunger? Caffeine naturally has the ability to make you feel satiated or "full" when consumed. It also helps with the mobilization of fatty acids in the body, meaning it helps move stored fatty acids into the mitochondria, turning it into energy, therefore giving you more energy. Having more energy will help you stay productive and distracted throughout your fast.

Green Tea: Let's take a quick look at green teas: Green tea can help decrease the hormone responsible for hunger in our bodies, called Ghrelin. When fasting, it's better you steep green tea in a water bottle overnight in the fridge. (Big Lean tip) When you wake up in the morning, drink the whole bottle before breaking your fast. This can help you feel more energized without feeling hungry throughout the morning.

4. Try Sugar-Free Diet Sodas, Flavored water (sugar free) andSugarless gum

There's no evidence so far pointing that artificial sweeteners are bad for health so definitely give these a try if nothing else works and with moderation it should be fine.

5. Try a Tablespoon or Two of Psyllium Husk

Psyllium husk is a fiber supplement that helps massively with hunger, and it signals to your brain that you have food in your digestive system.

6. Brush Your Teeth

This has been proven to reduce the feeling of hunger.

7. Keep Yourself Active and Flowing

Do something you enjoy, and immerse yourself in activities especially during that morning period when you're most productive.

6-7 hours fly by very fast when you're in the state of flow.

If you don't have more work to do go for a short walk while listening to an audiobook.

By doing that you'll burn some extra fat, and learn more.

This is opposite of what most people are doing by putting themselves in a low consciousness zombie mode with TV and Social Media .

And we all know people eat because they're bored.

Stay busy, stay productive.

8. Get Enough Sleep

Shortened sleep time is associated with decreases in leptin and elevations in ghrelin which means more hunger.

A study comparing 2 groups that were on a 700 calorie daily deficit with 2 different sleep duration found that:

The 8.5 hour group lost about 50/50 fat and lean mass. The 5.5 hour group lost 20/80 fat and lean mass.

Research also found that:

"If you get 6 hours of sleep per night for two weeks straight, your mental and physical performance declines to the same level as if you had stayed awake for 48 hours straight."

As you can see sleep is absolutely critical not just for intermittent fasting but for everything in your life.

9. Drink tones of water!

The average person should be drinking around 2 LITERS of water a day, and most of us don't even get CLOSE to that! Drinking the right amount of water is super important for our bodies to function properly. When we are dehydrated, we can tend to feel low in energy, tired and HUNGRY. That's right! You have probably heard it before, but our bodies don't have "as clear" of a signal to tell us that we need more water (sometimes a headache), so instead, we feel HUNGRY, when really it is WATER that we need! Drinking tons of water during our fast can not only help us avoid feeling hungry, but it will also help keep us hydrated and feeling GOOD! During a fast, you have the opportunity to really monitor your water intake, making sure you are staying hydrated with the proper amount of water!

10. Carbonated water

Carbonated water can be a GREAT help when you are feeling hungry during a fast. Any plain carbonated water or 0 calorie sweetened carbonated waters are safe to drink while fasting (ex. Le Croix, Bubbly). Carbonated water can make you feel more full than regular water because it contains carbon dioxide! Carbon dioxide fills up your tummy super fast and can really help if you are having intense food cravings.

In conclusion, hunger during IF is only an issue for the first few weeks until your body gets used to the new schedule.

And the ideas I've outlined here will get you through those hard times. Now, most people are not hungry anymore 4-8 weeks into intermittent fasting. So it's safe to say that the hardest period is the first 2-3 weeks.

And to be fair if you don't notice improvements after 4 weeks then maybe IF isn't for you. Research scientists agree that it's not a universal must-do approach for everyone.

What to drink: Practising intermittent fasting for weight loss

1.Tea

If you are a tea lover, you will be happy to know that this hot drink goes hand in hand with the goals of intermittent fasting. Here are its benefits:

- **It helps reduce hunger**

It's a big point! When we do not eat as much as usual, we are hungry! This is due to an imbalance of the hormone of hunger, ghrelin. We must go back to this balance if we want to feel less hunger.

Catechins present in green tea, among others, have the effect of regulating the level of ghrelin in the body.

Otherwise, the amount of ghrelin will naturally decrease over time. The less you eat, the less ghrelin is produced.

- **It helps with weight loss**

Different teas can positively influence weight loss.

a) Catechins found in green tea burn visceral body fat, which happens to be the fat around the abdomen. Storing this type of fat can increase the risk of insulin resistance and type 2 diabetes.

b) Other studies have shown that white tea is just as effective as green tea inburning visceral fat.

c) The combination of catechins and caffeine in green and white teas helpsto activate the metabolism, up to 4% in some cases. Having a good metabolism helps to burn more calories during the day.

2.Coffee

This contains caffeine, which increases alertness and helps curb appetite. Besides, caffeine also boosts metabolism and aids weight loss.

Therefore, drinking coffee is a great idea to control hunger and burn more fat while you are fasting.

3.Apple Cider Vinegar (ACV)

Apple cider vinegar contains mostly water and acids such as acetic acid and malic acid. 15 ml (one tablespoon) of apple cider vinegar contains approximately 3 calories. Perfect for weightloss!

What to drink: Practising intermittent fasting for autophagy

Autophagy is a process of the human body that consists of destroying old damaged cells. If these cells remain in the body, they cause inflammation which then leads to other health problems.

The intermittent fasting already stimulates autophagy, helping to cleanse the body.

Green tea - contains active polyphenols such as epigallocatechin gallate (EGCG) as well as caffeine, all combined giving an extra boost to autophagy!

Bone Broth - Combining broth drinking with intermittent fasting leaves you with glowing skin, better hair and nails, reduced inflammation and a slowed aging process.

It doesn't matter if your goal is to lose weight or to generally improve your health – bone broth is a must in your diet.

Who should not practise intermittent fasting?

- Women who want to get pregnant, are pregnant, or are breastfeeding.
- Those who are malnourished or underweight.
- Children under 18 years of age and elders.
- Those who have gout.
- Those who have gastroesophageal reflux disease (GERD).
- Those who have eating disorders should first consult with their doctors.
- Those who are taking diabetic medications and insulin must first consult with their doctors as dosages will need to be reduced.
- Those who are taking medications should first consult with their doctors as the timing of medications may be affected.
- Those who feel very stressed or have cortisol issues should not fast because fasting is another stressor.

- Those who are training very hard most days of the week should not fast.

IF for women over 50 years?

Obviously our bodies and our metabolism changes when we hit menopause. One of the biggest changes that women over 50 experience is that they have a slower metabolism and they start to put on weight. Fasting may be a good way to reverse and prevent this weight gain though. Studies have shown that this fasting pattern helps to regulate appetite and people who follow it regularly do not experience the same cravings that others do. If you're over 50 and trying to adjust to your slower metabolism, intermittent fasting can help you to avoid eating too much on a daily basis.

When you reach 50, your body also starts to develop some chronic diseases like high cholesterol and high blood pressure. Intermittent fasting has been shown to decrease both cholesterol and blood pressure, even without a great deal of weight loss. If you've started to notice your numbers rising at the doctor's office each year, you may be able to bring them back down with fasting, even without losing much weight.

Intermittent fasting may not be a great idea for every woman. Anyone with a specific health condition or who tends to be hypoglycemic should consult with a doctor. However, this new dietary trend has specific benefits for women who naturally store more fat in their bodies and may have trouble getting rid of these fat stores.

CHAPTER FIVE

How to excercise safely during intermittent fasting

The success of any weight loss or exercise program depends on how safe it is to sustain over time. If your ultimate goal is to decrease body fat and maintain your fitness level while doing IF, you need to stay in the safe zone. Here are some expert tips to help you do just that.

Eat a meal close to your moderate - to high-intensity workout

This is where meal timing comes into play. Khorana says that timing a meal close to a moderate- or high-intensity workout is key. This way your body has some glycogen stores to tap into to fuel your workout.

-Stay hydrated

Sonpal says to remember fasting doesn't mean to remove water. In fact, he recommends that you drink more water while fasting.

-Keep your electrolytes up

A good low-calorie hydration source, says Sonpal, is coconut water. "It replenishes electrolytes, is low in calories and tastes pretty good," he says. Gatorade and sports drinks are high in sugar, so avoid drinking too much of them.

-Keep the intensity and duration fairly low

If you push yourself too hard and begin to feel dizzy or light-headed, take a break. Listening to your body is important.

-Consider the type of fast

If you're doing a 24-hour intermittent fast, Lippin says you should stick to low-intensity workouts such as walking, restorative yoga, or gentle pilates. But if you're doing the 16:8 fast, much of the 16-hour fasting window is evening, sleep, and early in the day, so sticking to a certain type of exercise isn't as critical.

-Listen to your body

The most important advice to heed when exercising during IF is to listen to your body. "If you start to feel weak or dizzy, chances are you're experiencing low blood sugar or are dehydrated," explains Amengual. If that's the case, she says to opt for a carbohydrate-electrolyte drink immediately and then follow up with a well-balanced meal.

While exercising and intermittent fasting may work for some people, others may not feel comfortable doing any form of exercise while fasting. Check with your doctor or healthcare provider before starting any nutrition or exercise program.

Train your body into a fat-burning machine

I advise that you do it gradually or you may be tempted to quit when your body is not given enough time to adjust. You will need to remove or reduce carbohydrate intake to the bare minimum in order to trigger this. Once your body has no glycogen to burn, it will tap into your fat storage to burn fat. This process is called ketogenesis. This process produces ketones into our blood, which are then used as energy.

Ketones produce much more powerful energy. They do not send our insulin level into a roller-coaster ride.

Some of the symptoms when you have entered into ketosis mode are:

- You will soon notice the difference when your body is adapted to fat burning mechanism
- You will notice a new-found energy that has not been activated for a very long time
- You will notice that your mind is clearer and has much better focus
- No mid-afternoon sleepiness
- You will be able to control your physical hunger.

I advise you to quit the following to ease the transition.

Sugar

The bad news just keeps on coming for people who love sugar in their diet. We are now aware of the difficulties that sugar can bring to our insulin levels, and with diabetes becoming more prevalent physical health issues caused by it are also becoming more common. Sugar can make food taste good and people can become addicted to it, but it is a product we would all do well to keep under 25 grams a day, and even less if we already have insulin issues.

But now sugar is becoming linked with mental health issues, particularly Alzheimer's disease and other dementia problems. These issues are becoming more and more evident in our society and once we have acquired these problems they are often difficult to control, much less eliminate. So what are the ways in which sugar, this poison that we put too much of in our system, can affect our mental health? In at least a couple of ways actually, and we will describe them here.

1. The brain and glucose. Some defenders of sugar have said that at leastyou need some glucose because that's what your brain runs on. Some experts are now under the belief that the brain fires on glucose only because that is all that's available, and when it does we are finding that it damages the brain structure and function.

The really healthy fuels for the brain are other types of fuels, and particularly ketones, which the body produces when digesting healthy fats. In one test of healthy seniors who didn't suffer from any kind of dementia, higher levels of glucose were associated with poor memory, and the hippocampus structure of the brain was compromised. The shrinking of the hippocampus is considered a long-term precursor for Alzheimer's disease.

2. The liver and sugar, and what it all means for our brain. An essentialbuilding block for optimal brain function is cholesterol, which is produced in our liver. Our hard-working liver has many functions, and this is an important one, but also one of its critical functions is processing sugar. By increasing the task of processing fructose the liver has less time to produce what the brain really needs, which is that vital cholesterol.

We know that the brain has great adaptability, and by choosing a good diet, exercising regularly and opting for generally good lifestyle choices we can avoid many of the problems associated with old age. But in doing this we are pretty much on our own for maintaining the needed discipline. There is an entire industry promoting sugar and other processed foods, telling us that these dangerous toxic substances are actually good for us.

Other Dangers Include

- **Heart Threat** - Sugar has been shown to affect the involuntary muscle activity of the heart. A molecule found in ordinary table sugar called G6P has a negative impact on heart tissue at the cellular level.

Excess consumption of sugar and a sedentary lifestyle can increase a person's risk of developing heart failure. Heart failure often claims peoples lives in less than a decade after diagnosis.

- **Belly Fat** - There has been an alarming rise in obesity rates in teenagers and small children over these past few decades. One of the major contributing factors to this trend is an increase in the consumption of fructose. Fructose is an inexpensive form of sugar used in soda, ice cream, cookies and even bread products.

Fructose appears to boost the growth of visceral fat or the fat found in our midsections. When a child develops mature visceral fat early in life, he/she has a higher risk of being obese in adulthood.

- **Deadly Appetite -** Our bodies are naturally equipped with mechanisms that tell us when to stop eating. Studies show that sugar has found a way to suspend those natural mechanisms. Consuming foods and beverages rich in sugar contributes to the development of a condition called leptin resistance.

When a person has leptin resistance they don't feel full and satisfied with moderate amounts of food, so they continue consuming excessive amounts of food every time they eat.

Our bodies also have a tough time detecting the presence of sugar in beverages. It's difficult for the body to send a signal that you already consumed a lot of calories from soda or juices because this substance just doesn't register the same way as other types of food.

- Reduces our natural defense against bacterial defense (infectious disease) Leads to cancer
- Weakens eyesight
- Causes hypoglycemia and diabetes
- Causes a rapid adrenaline levels rise in children
- Causes premature aging
- Contributes to obesity
- Increases the risk of Crohn's disease

- Causes arthritis
- Causes asthma
- Causes gallstones
- Causes heart disease
- Causes hemorrhoids
- Causes varicose veins
- Decreases growth hormones
- Increases cholesterol
- Interferes with the absorption of protein
- Causes food allergies
- Causes cataracts
- Ages our skin
- Increases the size of our liver and kidneys
- Makes tendons more brittle
- Causes headaches and migraines
- Increases the risk of getting gout
- Can contribute to Alzheimer's disease
- Causes dizziness

Is addictive

Withdrawal effects of q uitting sugar

It took me about a year to consciously remove sugar from my diet. Once you have gone through that, you will live with so much energy without craving sugary food.

When you significantly slash your sugar intake, it can cause your blood sugar to drop, which can result in a host of symptoms as your body starts to adapt to finding new sources of energy. Sugar withdrawal nausea, headaches and fatigue are just a few of the typical side effects many report as a result of sugar withdrawal.

Of course, the severity of your symptoms largely depends on the amount of sugar in your diet beforehand. If you were loading up on the candy and sweet treats before, you're more likely to experience some of these symptoms than if sugar made up only a small part of your diet previously.

Some Of The Most Common Symptoms Caused By Sugar Withdrawal Include:

- Headaches
- Bloating
- Nausea
- Muscle aches
- Diarrhea
- Fatigue
- Hunger
- Anxiety
- Depression
- Cravings
- Chills

SUGAR WITHDRAWAL STAGES

Although the list of common side effects can be a bit daunting, keep in mind that these symptoms are temporary and generally only last a few days for most people. Here are the stages you can expect to encounter when you decide to drop sugar from your diet:

1. Feeling Motivated

When you make the decision to kick sugar to the curb, you will likely feel highly motivated and ready to reap the rewards of a healthier diet and lifestyle. Keep it up, as you'll need this motivation to propel you through the cravings, headaches and fatigue yet to come.

2. Cravings Start to Kick In

Cravings are one of the earliest signs of sugar withdrawal. Many people, for instance, establish a routine with their diets, and may find themselves glancing over at the vending machine when that mid-morning hunger starts to set in.

During this phase it's best to prepare by keeping healthy snacks at hand so it's even easier to resist the urge to indulge in your favorite sweets.

3. Symptoms Peak

Soon after the cravings hit, you may begin to experience some of the previously mentioned sugar withdrawal symptoms. Headaches, hunger, chills and even sugar withdrawal diarrhea can set in and make it harder than ever to stay motivated.

Remember why you decided to start eating more healthily and use that to keep you driven and determined to stay on the path to better health.

4. You Start to Feel Better

Once your symptoms start to clear up, you'll likely find yourself feeling better than ever. Many people have reported improvements in skin health, reduced brain fog and a boost in energy levels as a result of giving up added sugar.

Plus, by following a healthy diet and including more nutrient-dense foods in your day, you'll enjoy a lower risk of chronic disease and better overall health as well.

HOW TO REDUCE SUGAR CRAVINGS

First of all, do not try to cut yourself off from sugar altogether. While it may be tempting to cut it all out at once, this is a sure recipe for giving up and relapsing. Instead, try cutting one or two sugary foods out of your diet at a time. If you love soda, cookies, and a nightly bowl of ice cream, choose one of these at a time and find a healthier replacement. Instead of soda, try drinking fruit tea or water with a splash of fruit juice. If you love cookies, try making them yourself or eating fruit instead. If you wonder what you would do without your nightly bowl of ice cream, try a small square of organic dark chocolate instead. With substitutions like these, you will find it easier and easier to manage your sugar cravings without turning to processed sweets.

Once you've started controlling or eliminating the obvious sugars in your diet, start looking for the hidden sugars that you don't realize you are consuming. Make a habit of reading the label of everything that you purchase. You will be surprised at how many foods contain sugar or corn syrup as ingredients, even if they are not naturally sweet.

Making a conscious choice to purchase foods without added sugars is an excellent way to conquer your sugar cravings and reduce the amount of sugar that you are consuming.

If you still find yourself craving sugar, the next thing to try is a distraction. Strenuous exercise will help to distract you from your sugar cravings. As an added bonus exercise releases endorphins, which mimic the "high" that you get from eating sugary food but in a healthy way. Besides this, most people are reluctant to counteract the calorie burning effects of a strenuous workout with a pint of high fat ice cream.

Lastly, remember to give yourself a break. Allow yourself one healthy sweet per day. This could be a square of organic dark chocolate, a small bowl of natural ice cream, or even a piece of fruit that you've been saving. Reminding yourself that you have a treat waiting at home is an excellent way to motivate yourself to resist the sugar cravings that plague you as you are going through your daily routine.

DIFFERENT CHEMICAL ALTERNATIVE NAMES OF SUGAR

Sugar smells sweet and tastes sweet, but what about its name? How many sugar names are there? How many definitions? We use sugar to mean so many things, and food manufacturers often use it to disguise how bad the food is that we are eating.

"What's in a name? That which we call a rose by any other name would smell as sweet."

Added sugar goes by many names, and most types consist of glucose and/or fructose. High-fructose added sugars are more harmful.

1. Sugar/Sucrose

Sucrose is the most common type of sugar.

Often called "table sugar," it is a naturally occurring carbohydrate found in many fruits and plants.

Table sugar is usually extracted from sugar cane or sugar beets. It consists of 50% glucose and 50% fructose, bound together.

Sucrose is found in many foods, including ice cream, candy, pastries, cookies, soda, fruit juices, canned fruit, processed meat, breakfast cereals and ketchup, to name a few.

2. High-Fructose Corn Syrup (HFCS)

High-fructose corn syrup is a widely used sweetener, especially in the US.

It is produced from corn starch via an industrial process and consists of both fructose and glucose.

There are several different types of HFCS, which contain varying amounts of fructose.

Two notable varieties are:

- HFCS 55: This is the most common type of HFCS. It contains 55% fructose and 45% glucose, which makes it similar to sucrose in composition.
- HFCS 90: This form contains 90% fructose.

High-fructose corn syrup is found in many foods, especially in the US. These include soda, breads, cookies, candy, ice cream, cakes, cereal bars and many others.

3. Agave Nectar

Agave nectar, also called agave syrup, is a very popular sweetener produced from the agave plant.

It is commonly used as a "healthy" alternative to sugar because it doesn't spike blood sugar levels as much as many other sugar varieties.

However, agave nectar contains about 70–90% fructose, and 10–30% glucose.

Given the harmful health effects of excess fructose consumption, agave nectar may be even worse for metabolic health than regular sugar.

It is used in many "health foods," such as fruit bars, sweetened yogurts and cereal bars.

4–37. Other Sugars With Glucose and Fructose

Most added sugars and sweeteners contain both glucose and fructose.

Here are a few examples:

- Beet sugar
- Blackstrap molasses
- Brown sugar
- Buttered syrup
- Cane juice crystals
- Cane sugar
- Caramel
- Carob syrup
- Castor sugar
- Coconut sugar
- Confectioner's sugar (powdered sugar)
- Date sugar
- Demerara sugar
- Evaporated cane juice
- Florida Crystals
- Fruit juice
- Fruit juice concentrate
- Golden sugar
- Golden syrup
- Grape sugar
- Honey
- Icing sugar

Invert sugar

- Maple syrup
- Molasses
- Muscovado sugar
- Panela sugar
- Raw sugar
- Refiner's syrup
- Sorghum syrup
- Sucanat
- Treacle sugar
- Turbinado sugar

Yellow sugar

38–52. Sugars With Glucose

These sweeteners contain glucose, either pure or combined with sugars other than fructose (such as other glucose units or galactose):

- Barley malt
- Brown rice syrup
- Corn syrup
- Corn syrup solids
- Dextrin
- Dextrose
- Diastatic malt
- Ethyl maltol
- Glucose
- Glucose solids
- Lactose
- Malt syrup
- Maltodextrin
- Maltose

Rice syrup

53–54. Sugars With Fructose Only

These two sweeteners contain only fructose:

- Crystalline fructose
- Fructose

55–56. Other Sugars

There are a few added sugars that contain neither glucose nor fructose. They are less sweet and less common, but are sometimes used as sweeteners:

- D-ribose
- Galactose

There was nothing that i enjoyed much more than sipping a cup of Earl Grey with a spoonful of sugar. I used to drink that every weekend. I had to quit doing that considering the harm it did to my body. At this moment, I have no slight craving to drink tea (with sugar) anymore, and when a certain food contains a little sugar, I would be able to taste the sweetness when others may not taste the sweetness.

As parents of 3 years old boy, my wife and I were careful with the food intake of our son. Discouraging him from eating sweet food at a young age will make him less prone to develop a sweet tooth when he grows up. Our children are also exposed to sugary food at school. We can't control much with his food intake at school, i.e. we can't tell him not to eat his friend's birthday cake at school. We just do our part to control his food intake at home.

If you must take sugar, you can use xylitol instead, which has the lowest Glycemic Index and won't trigger insulin spike

Losing weight – Why calories loss counts

Over recent years, the focus in weight loss programs has been largely low carb or low fat diets. In order to lose weight, you need to eat fewer calories than you need to use across each day. So regardless of what your diet or eating program is called, the bottom line about all successful weight loss is calories loss.

Are you ready to figure out how many calories you should take in each day? There are several ways to decide what your ideal calorie intake should be. Some are complicated and involve calculating your Base Metabolic Rate and then adding the amount of energy you normally put into physical activity, and adding in how efficiently your body processes food.

You can go to a nutritionist who has tools to measure those values and get a very precise figure of how many calories you should be eating each day. But if you want a simpler formula to figure out how many calories you should be taking in each day to keep your body functioning, there is an easier way.

First, you need to assess your activity level.

You are sedentary if you sit at a computer all day and do no more physical activity than walking around the grocery store. The best way to figure out how many calories you need to take in on a daily basis is to take your weight and multiply it by 14, so if you weigh 150 pounds, you would multiply 150 x 14 and get 2100, so you need to take in 2,100 calories each day to maintain your weight. To lose weight through calories loss your intake will need to be less than this.

If you are moderately active, you don't work out every day but you might hit the gym two or three times a week or walk or bike ride around the neighborhood at night. To figure out how many calories you need each day, take your weight and multiply it by 17 so the total will give you the number of calories you should take in to maintain your weight. To lose weight through calories loss your intake will need to be less than this.

If you bike to work, go to the gym every day, or run five miles at night, you are active. In order to figure out your ideal calorie intake, multiply your weight by 20 and that is how many calories your body needs to keep working efficiently. To lose weight through calories loss your intake will need to be less than this.

A food diary is a great way to get an accurate idea of how many calories you consume in a day and figure out how many calories are in each of the things that you ate that day. There are lots of commercially available calorie counting books that give the total number of calories for a lot of common foods and even fast foods. Using a food diary you can accurately count the calories in a fast food meal and determine what and how much you can eat in order to lose weight through calories loss.

Counting calories may take a little time at the outset, but it becomes a lot easier and will help you control what you eat so you can lose weight and keep it off forever.

How to count calories according to body weight

Your caloric intake is the most important factor in determining your weight. It comes down to how many calories you consume versus how many you burn. Both exercise and diet influence how effectively you burn calories. Whether your goal is to lose, gain or maintain weight, there is a method to calculate your daily calorie requirements. You will need to know your current level of physical activity, height and weight to use the equation.

1.**Weigh yourself.** Use a bathroom scale to determine your weight in pounds. A scale usually gives your weight in stones.

2.**Calculate your basic metabolic rate (BMR).** Your BMR is your resting metabolic rate, which is how active your metabolism is when you are not performing any physical activity, such as sleep. If you're a woman, use the following formula to calculate your BMR: 655 + (4.35 x weight in pounds) + (4.7 x height in inches) - (4.7 x age in years).

Use the following formula to calculate your BMR if you are a man: 66 + (6.23 x weight in pounds) + (12.7 x height in inches) - (6.8 x age in years). For example, a 23-year-old man who is 6 feet 2 inches tall, weighing 185 pounds, has a basic metabolic rate of 2,003.

3. **Multiply your BMR by the level of physical activity you get** . If you get little or no exercise, times your BMR by 1.2, and if you perform light exercise, such as walking one to three days a week, multiply your BMR by 1.375. For a moderate level of exercise, such as jogging three to five times a week, multiply your BMR by 1.55. And for those who are very active and exercise or engage in sports most days of the week, times your BMR by 1.725. Calculate an athletic level of exercise by multiplying your BMR by 1.9. The result is the ideal number of calories you should consume daily. The very active 23-year-old man in the example above would multiply his BMR by 1.725, for a total of 3,452 calories daily.

4.Increase your ideal number of calories by 500 to 1,000 daily to increase your weight by 1 to 2 pounds a week, or decrease your calories if you want to lose weight.

Things You Will Need

- Scale
- Calculator
- Tip

Read nutrition labels or use an online calorie counter to find out the amount of calories in each meal you consume. This will help you keep track of your caloric intake.

CHAPTER SIX: Combining Intermittent Fasting and Ketogenic Diet

If you commit to the ketogenic diet while doing intermittent fasting as well, it could offer the following benefits.

-May Smooth Your Path to Ketosis

Intermittent fasting may help your body reach ketosis quicker than using the keto diet alone.

That's because your body, when fasting, maintains its energy balance by shifting its fuel source from carbs to fats — the exact premise of the keto diet.

During fasting, insulin levels and glycogen stores decrease, leading your body to naturally start burning fat for fuel.

For anyone who struggles to reach ketosis while on a keto diet, adding intermittent fasting may effectively jumpstart your process.

-May Lead to More Fat Loss

Combining the diet and the fast may help you burn more fat than the diet alone.

Because intermittent fasting boosts your metabolism by promoting thermogenesis, or heat production, your body may start utilizing stubborn fat stores.

Several studies have revealed that intermittent fasting can powerfully and safely drop excess body fat.

In an eight-week study in 34 resistance-trained men, those who practiced the 16/8 method of intermittent fasting lost nearly 14% more body fat than those following a normal eating pattern.

Similarly, a review of 28 studies noted that people who used intermittent fasting lost an average of 7.3 pounds (3.3 kg) more fat mass than those following very low-calorie diets.

Plus, intermittent fasting may preserve muscle mass during weight loss and improve energy levels, which may be helpful for keto dieters looking to improve athletic performance and drop body fat.

Additionally, studies underscore that intermittent fasting can reduce hunger and promote feelings of fullness, which may aid weight loss.

Combining the ketogenic diet with intermittent fasting is likely safe for most people.

However, pregnant or breastfeeding women and those with a history of disordered eating should avoid intermittent fasting.

People with certain health conditions, such as diabetes or heart disease, should consult with a doctor before trying intermittent fasting on the keto diet.

Though some people may find merging the practices helpful, it's important to note that it may not work for everyone.

Some people may find that fasting on the keto diet is too difficult, or they may experience adverse reactions, such as overeating on non-fasting days, irritability and fatigue.

Keep in mind that intermittent fasting is not necessary to reach ketosis, even though it can be used as a tool to do so quickly.

Simply following a healthy, well-rounded keto diet is enough for anyone looking to improve health by cutting down on carbs.

Smoothies for keto

You may be one of those people who has made the decision to lead a healthier lifestyle. Is that why you are looking for a bit of help? Are you here because you want to know more about how to make delicious and spectacular smoothies?

Smoothie information is so in-demand these days. But what makes smoothies special when they are just part purée and part fruit drink? They are easy to make, so much so that anyone can prepare one. It takes no special skill to concoct a foamy, fruity mix that you can enjoy by yourself or share with people close to you.

What makes smoothies a special type of beverage is that they can be so nutritious that you won't need to take multivitamins and other expensive supplements anymore if you include smoothies in your daily diet. Smoothies are very good for you.

There was a time when smoothies were novelties and specialities offered only in cafes, restaurants, and juice bars. Now you can make them at home. If you are new to the smoothie phenomenon, you can learn how to make a handful of basic preparations such as strawberry smoothies, banana smoothies, and mango smoothies. But you should realize that there is a whole new world of smoothie information that you have not yet glimpsed. Allow us to impart a few tips that you can use to make more refreshing, exciting, and very delicious smoothie preparations.

Smoothies are first and foremost an excellent way to get healthy. They allow you to meet your daily recommended servings of fruits and vegetables that many people lack in their diets. Smoothies allow you to create a drink using whole fruits and vegetables without discarding much of the fruit or vegetables as you would do if you ate the fruit or vegetable itself.

Benefits of smoothies

Smoothies aren't only beverages that go with the new trend. They give benefits which are good to health at the same time.

Here are some benefits that smoothies contain:

1. **Milk-Based Smoothies Provide Calcium -** Smoothies that were made with dairy products give calcium for bone strength so that they will stay strong even into old age. Whole milk gives almost a third of your daily requirements of calcium. It also contains fats and vitamins to keep our body alive.

2. **Smoothies Make A Healthy Breakfast More Convenient -** A homemade smoothie for your morning meal is excellent. It gives you energy to maintain cheerfulness until the end of the day. Drinking a smoothie in the morning helps you stop indulging in empty carbohydrates. In fact, a nutritious smoothie does better when it comes to body enrichment that multivitamins do.

3. **Good Smoothies Are Nutrient- Dense and Contain Fat -** the best smoothies are nutrient - dense, providing vitamins and oils necessary for good nutrition. Fat is required for biological function and is burned by your body for energy; it also helps with the maintenance of our body.

4. **Healthy Smoothies Are Simple To Make -** Healthy smoothies are easy to produce. When you have a good blender and quality ingredients, you can now have a delicious, healthy smoothie in just a snap. It's not the thing that would consume a great amount of time but it helps you to create an instant but healthy beverage.

5. **Smoothies Help You Keep Hydrated -** A smoothie for breakfast helps you keep hydrated at the start of the day. A glass of smoothie will quench your thirst so you don't have to drink water every time you get thirsty.

Making and drinking these smoothies is a good habit for every day and is a great replacement for sodas and any other forms of beverages which don't have positive nutritional effects on the body.

Basic components of a smoothie

If you're going to try your hand at making your own smoothies, there are a few things you need to know. Smoothie ingredients break down into three categories: fruit, liquid and additions. Let's look at each of these in turn.

First, let's talk about fruit. Fruit forms the foundation of your smoothie. The fruit flavor will usually dominate, so you can pick your favorite fruits to give your smoothie its primary flavour identity. Now, not all fruit actually works in smoothies. Some fruits do well, others do horribly.

Creamy fruits, berries and stone fruits like peaches all work well in smoothies. Melons can work well in small amounts (or you can blend up a bunch of melon with other ingredients for one of your wilder smoothie experiments). However, lots of popular fruits don't work particularly well in smoothies. Apples, for instance, don't really make great smoothie foundation material. Use apple cider as a liquid base instead for an appleflavoured smoothie.

Since there are so many different types of fruits, I can't really tell you which ones will work and which ones won't on a case by case basis. Just be aware that some of the fruits you add to your smoothies might not actually end up working well. And that's totally okay.

Once you've chosen your fruit, you need to add in a liquid. Juices work really well. Water tends to be a little tricky because your smoothie can easily end up quite tasteless. It's weird how you can have tons of fruits and other ingredients, but water's dilutional power simply takes the edge off of all the flavors. My personal favorite (current) smoothie liquid is coconut water. You can find it at some health food stores, or do what I do and order it directly from Amazon for a discount.

Finally, no smoothie would be complete without some extra ingredients. This is where the sky really is the limit. You can add nutritional supplements (particularly the powdered kind), nuts (use raw nuts or be prepared to ruin your nut addition) and leafy greens (spinach, kale and parsley are fantastic but use these with care lest your smoothie be more nutritious than actually tasty).

How to make smoothies

Using The Right Equipment To Make The Perfect Smoothie

Most people prefer learning how to make smoothies with a good quality smoothie blender. While there are cheaper ones available in the market, they have limited functions. A marvelous blender will allow you to make the best smoothies with just the right texture.

Ingredients To Li q uefy Your Smoothie

There are a few basic building blocks when it comes time to make a smoothie. The first essential ingredient is the liquid or thinning agent. Liquids like fresh milk, cow's milk, and soy milk are great options. These will offer you a dose of calcium, protein, and contains flavones. While fruit juices can also be used, they generally have a high sugar content and if your intention is to learn how to make smoothies that are nutritional, you would do better to skip the fruit juice and stick to soy milk instead.

Fresh Produce

To this liquid, you must add your choice of fruits and vegetables. These change the taste as well as the texture of your smoothie. Pick tastes that blend well together. You can keep mixing and matching to find the smoothie that you like best. In your journey of how to make smoothies that are delicious as well as healthy, feel free to use fruits like strawberries, blackberries, apples, kiwis, cherries, grapes, and vegetables like pumpkin, and raw spinach! These ingredients pack a powerful punch and are full of nutritional value.

Thickening Ingredient

The next step in learning how to make smoothies is to add a thickener to the mixture. This can be added in the form of ice crushed, cubes, and frozen fruit depending on the strength and capacity of your blender. Frozen fruits can also be used as a thickening agent but again you will need a powerful blender that will purify them. This ingredient adds to the texture and consistency of the smoothie.

While learning how to make smoothies, you need to realize that this is a process that is flexible and depends entirely on your taste and preferences. If you prefer your smoothies a little runny, consider using less of the thickener and more of the milk or juice. If the smoothies turn out to be too thin, simply add more frozen fruits or ice. If you feel like your smoothie is too watered down, add some more fruit to it. If you want to add a little more flavor to it, add some cinnamon or honey.

To achieve the right consistency, most blenders take within 30 to 45 seconds to fully chop up or blend the ingredients. Allow your smoothie to circulate freely without any lumps inside the blender for at least 5 to 10 seconds before you consider it ready. Now you've learned how to make smoothies!

Since each of those three categories contains a near-infinite potential for variation, you can see that the number of total smoothies is basically infinite. Don't be afraid to mix up something strange! Instead, be brave, get out your blender and have at it--it's smoothie time!

Smoothie recipes for weight loss

Many people wonder if the smoothie diet will work to help them lose weight. If you follow the right plan, the weight can come off pretty darn quick for you too.

The smoothie method for losing weight is essentially a low-calorie diet where you substitute your usual meals with fruit or vegetable smoothies.

For smoothie enthusiasts - let me tell you - when you do this, it will not feel like you are dieting at all. You will not feel deprived as you do on most diets.

And if you do it right you won't suffer from those awful hunger pains. This is not a starvation diet - this is a healthy, nutritious, delicious meal replacement diet that you do short term to supercharge weight loss and flood your body with living foods that give you lots of nutrition and vitamins.

So how does drinking smoothies help you lose weight? Smoothies, when made correctly and nutritiously, can fill you up so you are NOT hungry and you won't be tempted to eat forbidden high-calorie foods.

Can you lose weight fast? It depends.... if you follow the wrong plan you may end up drinking smoothies that are high calorie and low in nutritional value. You know, it is the same way that you can ruin a healthy salad by pouring half a container of high-fat dressing on it. With this in mind, I've put together these simple, healthy recipes for weight loss that will have you on your way to dropping those pounds quickly.

These recipes will not only allow you to feel full during fasting, but are also suitable for weightloss.

1. Low Carb Acai Almond Butter Smoothie

Servings: 1

Ingredients:

- 1 100g pack unsweetened acai puree
- 3/4 cup unsweetened almond milk
- 1/4 of an avocado
- 3 tbsp collagen or protein powder
- 1 tablespoon coconut oil or MCT oil powder
- 1 tablespoon almond butter
- 1/2 teaspoon vanilla extract
- 2 drops liquid stevia (optional) *Instructions:*

- If you are using individualized 100 gram packs of acai puree, run the pack under lukewarm water for a few seconds until you are able to break up the puree into smaller pieces. Open the pack and put the contents into the blender.

- Place the remaining ingredients in the blender and blend until smooth. Add more water or ice cubes as needed.
- Drizzle the almond butter along the side of the glass to make it look cool.
- Enjoy and pat yourself on the back for an awesome workout and killer post workout smoothie!

Nutritional Values:

- Calories: 345 Kcal
- Fat: 20g
- Carbohydrates: 8g
- Fiber: 2g
- Protein: 15g

2. Keto Blueberry Smoothie

Servings: 1

This keto smoothie is perfect for a quick breakfast or a post-workout refuel option. It's packed with antioxidants for better detoxification, Vitamin C for a healthy immune system, and folate for proper cholesterol function.

Ingredients:

- 1 cup coconut milk or almond milk
- 1/4 cup blueberries
- 1 tsp vanilla extract
- 1 tsp MCT oil or coconut oil
- 30 g protein powder (optional)

Instructions:

- Put all the ingredients into a blender, and blend until smooth.

Notes

If you like the swirl, you can add a tablespoon of full-fat yogurt after the smoothie is in the cup and swirl it around, touching the sides.

Suitable Substitutions

MCT Oil - If you don't have any MCT oil that's totally fine, you can replace this with coconut oil or any fat you like.

Blueberries - Any berry will work (blackberry, raspberry, strawberry) and will have a similar carbohydrate content.

Protein Powder - If you don't have protein powder, you can simply omit this from the recipe. If you still want a fluffy texture you could try adding a raw egg, but these can sometimes contain salmonella so pregnant women should avoid this.

Milk Alternatives - you can make this with unsweetened almond milk, unsweetened coconut milk, pea milk, and they all taste similar; just find milk you like, and use that.

Nutritional Values:

- Calories: 215 Kcal

- Fat: 10g
- Carbohydrates: 7g
- Fiber: 3g
- Protein: 23g

3. Minty Green Protein Smoothie (Dairy Free & Low Carb)

Servings: 1

Ingredients:

- 1/2 of an avocado
- 1 cup fresh spinach
- 10-12 drops SweetLeaf® Liquid Stevia Peppermint Sweet Drops™
- 1 scoop Whey Protein Powder
- 1/2 cup unsweetened almond milk
- 1/4 teaspoon peppermint extract
- 1 cup ice
- Optional: cacao nibs

Instructions:

- Place avocado, spinach, protein powder and milk in a blender and blend until smooth. Add the SweetLeaf® Liquid Stevia Peppermint Sweet Drops™, extract, and ice, and blend until thick. Taste and adjust stevia, as needed.

Nutritional Values:

- Net carbs: 4g
- Calories: 293 Kcal
- Fat: 15g
- Fiber: 7g
- Protein: 28

4. Turmeric Keto Smoothie

Servings: 1

Ingredients:

- 200 ml full fat coconut milk
- 200 ml unsweetened almond milk
- 1 teaspoon granulated sweetener (stevia etc.) or other sweetener
- 1 tablespoon ground turmeric
- 1 teaspoon ground cinnamon
- 1 teaspoon ground ginger
- 1 tbsp MCT oil or use coconut oil
-

1 tablespoon chia seeds to top *Instructions:*

- Combine all the ingredients except the chia seeds in a blender, add some ice and blend until smooth.
- Sprinkle chia seeds on top and enjoy!

Nutritional Values:

- Fat: 56g
- Protein: 7g
- Net Carbs: 6g
- Calories: 600 Kcal

5. Raspberry Avocado Smoothie - Dairy Free

Servings: 2

Ingredients:

- 1 ripe avocado, peeled and with pit removed
- 1 1/3 cup water
- 2-3 tablespoons lemon juice
- 2 tbsp low carb sugar substitute - I like to use 1/8 teaspoon liquid stevia extract
- 1/2 cup frozen unsweetened raspberries or other low carb frozen berries

Instructions:

- Add all ingredients to blender.
- Blend until smooth.
- Pour into two tall glasses and enjoy with a straw!

Nutritional Values per serving:

- Net carbs: 4g
- Calories: 227 kcal
- Fat: 20g
- Fiber: 8.8g
- Protein: 2.5g

6. Mean Green Matcha Protein Shake

Matcha powder, protein powder, almond milk, and leafy greens make up this matcha protein shake. Have it as a breakfast smoothie or a pre-workout snack for the energy boost you crave.

Servings: 1

Ingredients:

- 1 cup unsweetened milk of choice
- ¼ cup coconut milk
- 1 scoop Perfect Keto Unflavored Whey Protein Powder or vanilla protein powder
- 1 scoop Perfect Keto Matcha MCT oil powder
- 1 large handful spinach
- 1 small avocado
- 1 tablespoon coconut oil
- 1 cup of ice (optional)

Instructions:

- Add all ingredients to a high-speed blender and mix on high until smooth.

- Garnish with chopped mint leaves and a few berries if desired.

Nutritional Values:

- Calories: 334 Kcal
- Fat: 24g
- Carbohydrates: 13g
- Fiber: 10g
- Protein: 19g

7. Keto Beetroot Shake

Servings: 1

Ingredients:

- 1 tsp Temple Nutrition Beetroot Powder
- 1 tbsp Temple Nutrition MCT Oil (use 1 tsp if you are new to MCT oil)
- 1 scoop Whey Protein Isolate (Optional)
- 1 tsp vanilla extract
- 1/4 teaspoon cinnanmon, ground
- 1 cup coconut milk or almond milk, pea milk

Instructions:

- Put all ingredients into a high speed blender.
- Blend for 30 seconds.
- Pour into a glass, or drink straight from the container. Top with extra beetroot powder if desired.

Nutritional Values:

- Calories: 300 Kcal
- Fat: 19g
- Carbohydrates: 6g
- Fiber: 3g
- Protein 25g

Keto recipes

Keto breakfast recipes

1. Keto Coffee Recipe – 4 Variations

Prep Time: 2 Minutes

Cook Time: 5 Minutes

Servings: 1

Keto Coffee Recipe – Variation 1 – Traditional

Ingredients:

- 1 cup (240 ml) black coffee
- 1/2 teaspoon (2 ml) MCT oil (add more once you know you can handle it!)
- 1 Tablespoon (15 ml) ghee *Nutritional*

Values per serving:

- Calories: 143 Kcal
- Fat: 17g
- Net Carbs: 0g
- Protein: 0g

Keto Coffee Recipe – Variation 2 – Coconut

Ingredients:

- 1 cup (240 ml) of black coffee
- 1/2 Tablespoon (7 ml) coconut oil
- 1 Tablespoon (15 ml) ghee

Nutritional Values per serving:

Calories: 179 Kcal
Fat: 21g
Net Carbs: 0g
Protein: 0g

Keto Coffee Recipe – Variation 3 – Frothy

Ingredients:

- 1 cup (240 ml) of black coffee
- 1/2 Tablespoon (7 ml) coconut oil
- 1 Tablespoon (15 ml) ghee
- 2 Tablespoons (30 ml) unsweetened coconut or almond

milk*Nutritional Values per serving:*

- Calories: 190 Kcal
- Fat: 22g
- Net Carbs: 0g
- Protein: 0g

Keto Coffee Recipe – Variation 4 – Collagen Boosted

Ingredients:

- 1 cup (240 ml) of black coffee
- 1 Tablespoon (15 ml) ghee
-

- 1/2 scoop unflavored hydrolyzed collagen powder (try
- CoBionic Indulgence to add a mocha flavor to your coffee!)
- *Nutritional Values per serving:*
- Calories: 160 Kcal
- Fat: 14g
- Net Carbs: 0g
- Protein: 5g

Instructions:

-

Combine all ingredients in a blender. Pour into a coffee mug to serve.

2. Keto Chocolate Hazelnut Muffins Recipe (Dairy-Free)

Prep Time: 10 Minutes

Cook Time: 20 Minutes

Yield: 12 Muffins

Ingredients:

- 3 cups (360 g) almond flour
- 1/2 cup (120 ml) coconut oil, melted
- 4 large eggs, whisked
- 1/2 teaspoon nutmeg
- 1/4 teaspoon cloves
- 1/2 cup (100 g) hazelnuts, chopped
- Low carb sweetener of choice (we recommend Stevia), to taste
- Dash of salt
- 1 teaspoon (8 g) baking soda
- 3 oz (80 g) 100% dark chocolate, broken into chunks *Instructions:*

- Preheat oven to 350 F (175 C).
- Mix together the almond flour, coconut oil, eggs, nutmeg, cloves, chopped hazelnuts, sweetener, salt, and baking soda. Pour the
- mixture into 12 lined or greased muffin pans.
- Place chocolate chunks on the top each muffin, pressing them down into the dough/mixture.
- Bake for 18-20 minutes so that a toothpick comes out clean when you insert it into a muffin.

Nutritional Values per serving:

Serving Size: 1 muffin

-
-
-
-

- Calories: 282 Kcal

  Sugar: 1g
  Fat: 25g
  Carbohydrates: 6g
  Fiber: 3g
- Protein: 8g

3.Easy Breakfast Baked Egg in Avocado

Prep Time: 5 Minutes

Cook Time: 12 Minutes

Servings: 2

Ingredients:

- 1 avocado
- 2 egg yolks
- 2 teaspoons olive oil or coconut oil
- Salt and pepper and other seasoning/spices/herbs to taste

(smoked paprika goes well with eggs) *Instructions:*

- Preheat oven to 400 F (200 C).
- Slice the avocado in half and remove the stone.
- Crack the 2 eggs into a bowl.
- Scoop out each egg yolk and place each into an avocado half.
- Pour 1 teaspoon of olive oil onto each egg yolk in the avocado.
- Bake for 12 minutes.
- Sprinkle salt and pepper and whatever additional herbs and spices
- you'd like on top.

Nutritional Values per serving:

- Calories: 250 Kcal
- Sugar: 1g
  Fat: 23g

  Carbohydrates: 9g
  Fiber: 7g
  Protein: 3g

4. Keto Breakfast Stack

Prep Time: 15 Minutes

Cook Time: 15 Minutes

Servings: 2

Ingredients:

- 4 slices bacon (use AIP-compliant bacon if you're staying AIP)
- 1/4 lb (110 g) ground pork
- 1/4 lb (110 g) ground chicken
- 2 teaspoons (2 g) Italian seasoning
- 1 egg, whisked (omit for AIP)
- 1 teaspoon (5 g) salt
- 1/4 teaspoon black pepper (omit for AIP)
- 2 large flat mushrooms (like portobello)
- 1 avocado, sliced

Instructions:

- Cook the bacon until crispy. Leave the fat in the pan.

-
-
-
-

Mix together the ground pork, chicken, Italian seasoning, egg, salt, and pepper in a bowl and form 4 thin patties.

- Pan-fry the patties in the bacon fat.
- Then pan-fry the mushrooms.
- Put together your keto breakfast stack with the mushrooms on the bottom, then 2 thin patties, then 3 slices of avocado, and top it with the slices of bacon. Serve with the rest of the avocado slices.

Nutritional Values per serving:

Calories: 680 Kcal

Sugar: 2g
Fat: 54g
Carbohydrates: 13g
Fiber: 8g
- Protein: 38g

5. Paleo Chicken and Bacon Sausages

Prep Time: 10 Minutes

Cook Time: 20 Minutes

Servings: 12

Ingredients:

-

-
-
-

- 2 large chicken breasts, or use 1 lb ground chicken
- 2 slices bacon, cooked and broken into small bits
- 1 egg, whisked (omit for AIP)
- 2 tablespoons Italian seasoning
- 2 teaspoons garlic
-
- powder 2 teaspoons onion

powder Salt and pepper

Instructions:

- In a large skillet, melt the coconut oil over a medium-high heat. Add the turkey and bacon to the skillet and sauté until slightly browned – for about 5 to 7 minutes.
- Add the onion, asparagus, spinach and fresh thyme to the skillet. Sauté for an additional 10 minutes until the turkey and bacon are cooked through and the vegetables are soft.
- Season with salt and pepper, to taste.

Nutritional Values per serving:

- Calories: 370 Kcal
  Sugar: 1g

-

-
-
-

Fat: 21g
Carbohydrates: 3g
Fiber: 1g
- Protein: 40g

6. Almond Flour Pancakes (Keto-friendly)

Prep Time: 5 Minutes

Cook Time: 15 Minutes

Servings: 6

Ingredients:

- 1 cup blanched almond flour
- 2 eggs
- 2 tablespoons maple syrup (optional; or use water)
- 2 tablespoons olive oil (or any other liquid oil)
- 1 teaspoon baking powder
- 1 teaspoon vanilla extract
- 1/4 teaspoon fine sea salt

Instructions:

Skillet Pancakes:

- Preheat a skillet over a medium-low heat on the stove. As it heats, stir together the almond flour, eggs, maple syrup (if using), olive oil, baking powder, vanilla, and salt in a large bowl. The batter will be a little thicker than traditional pancake batter.
- Grease the preheated skillet with butter or olive oil, then pour 3 to 4 tablespoons of the batter into the center of the skillet (I use a scant 1/4

-

cup). Use a spatula to spread the batter out into a round pancake shape, about 1/4 to 1/2-inch thick.

- Cook until little bubbles start to form around the edges of the pancake, and as soon as the bottom feels sturdy enough to flip (about 3 to 4 minutes of cooking time), use a spatula to flip the pancake and cook the other side, about 2 to 3 more minutes.
  Repeat with the remaining batter, until all of the pancakes are cooked. I usually get about 6 pancakes from this batch that are roughly 4 to 6 inches in diameter. Even though they are on the smaller side, they are very filling! Serve warm with your favorite toppings.

Oven-Baked Pancakes:

- Prepare the batter as directed above, but instead of using the stove, preheat the oven to 350ºF and line a large baking sheet with parchment paper.
- Pour the prepared batter by a scant 1/4 cup onto the lined baking sheet, and use a spoon or spatula to spread the batter into a round pancake shape until it's 1/4-inch thick. Leave about 1 inch between each pancake, and repeat with the remaining batter until you have roughly 6 pancakes on the pan.
- Bake at 350ºF for 10 minutes. The pancakes should puff up, and you don't need to flip them as long as they look like they are thoroughly cooked through. I like to flip them over for serving, so the browned side is on top. Serve warm, with your favorite pancake toppings.

Nutrional values per serving:

Made with maple syrup:

- Calories: 193 Kcal
- Fat: 15g
- Carbohydrates: 9g
- Fiber: 1.5g
-

- Protein: 6g

Made without syrup:

- Calories: 175 Kcal
- Fat: 15g
- Carbohydrates: 4g
- Fiber: 1g

Protein: 6g

Keto lunch and dinner recipes

1. Bacon and Avocado Caesar Salad

Prep Time: 10 Minutes

Cook Time: 5 Minutes

Servings: 2

Ingredients:

For the salad:

- 4 slices of bacon (112 g), diced
- 1 head of romaine lettuce (200 g), chopped
- 1/2 cucumber (110 g), thinly sliced
- 1/4 medium onion (28 g), thinly sliced
- 1 large avocado (200 g), sliced

For the Caesar dressing:

-

- 1/4 cup of mayo (60 ml)
- 1 tablespoon of lemon juice (15 ml)
- 1 teaspoon of Dijon mustard (5 ml)
- 1 teaspoon of garlic powder (3.5
-

g) Salt and pepper, to taste *Instructions:*

- Add the bacon to a large nonstick skillet over medium-high heat and sauté until crispy, for about 5 minutes. Remove the bacon from the skillet with a slotted spoon and place on a paper towel lined plate to cool.
- In a small bowl, whisk to combine the mayo, lemon juice, mustard, and garlic powder. Season with salt and pepper, to taste.

- Toss the remaining Caesar dressing with the romaine lettuce leaves. Add the cucumber and onion to the bowl and toss to combine.
- Divide the salad between 2 plates and top each salad with equal amounts of cooked bacon and sliced avocado.

Nutritional Values per serving:

- Calories: 652 Kcal
- Sugar: 3g
- Fat: 65g
- Carbohydrates: 15g
- Fiber: 9g
- Protein: 10g

2.Lemon Garlic Ghee Keto Salmon Recipe with Leek Asparagus Ginger Saute

Prep Time: 10 Minutes

Cook Time: 20 Minutes

Servings: 2

Ingredients:

For the lemon garlic ghee salmon:

- 2 fillets of salmon (with skin on), fresh or frozen (340 g), defrost if frozen
- 1 tablespoon (15 ml) ghee (use avocado oil for AIP)
- 4 cloves garlic (12 g), minced
- 2 teaspoons (10 ml) lemon juice
- Salt to taste
- Lemon slices to serve with

For the leek asparagus ginger sauté:

- 10 spears of asparagus (160 g), chopped into small pieces
- 1 leek (90 g), chopped into small pieces

2 teaspoons (4 g) ginger powder (or use finely diced fresh ginger ifyou have it available)

- Avocado oil or olive oil to sauté with
- 1 Tablespoon lemon
- juice Salt to taste

Instructions:

- Preheat oven to 400 F (200 C).
- Place each salmon fillet on a piece of aluminum foil or parchment paper.
- Divide the ghee, lemon juice and minced garlic between the two fillets – place these on top of the salmon. Sprinkle with some salt. Then wrap up the salmon in the foil and place into the oven.
- Open up the foil after 10 minutes in the oven and then bake for another 10 minutes.
- While the salmon is cooking, place 1-2 tablespoons of avocado oil or olive oil into a frying pan and sauté the chopped asparagus and leek on a high heat. Saute for 10 minutes and then add in the ginger powder, lemon juice, and salt to taste. Saute for 1 more minute.
- Serve by dividing the sauté between 2 plates and placing a salmon fillet on top of each.

Nutritional Values per serving:

- Calories: 680 Kcal
- Sugar: 4g
- Fat: 51g
- Carbohydrates: 15g
- Fiber: 4g
- Protein: 4g

3. Lemon Black Pepper Tuna Salad Recipe

Prep Time: 10 Minutes

Cook Time: 0 Minutes

Servings: 1

Ingredients:

- 1/3 cucumber, diced small
- 1/2 small avocado, diced small
- 1 teaspoon lemon juice
- 1 can (4-6 oz or 100–150 g) of tuna
- 1 tablespoon Paleo mayo (use olive oil for AIP)
- 1 tablespoon mustard (omit for AIP)
- Salt to taste
- Salad greens (optional)
- Black pepper to taste (omit for AIP)

Instructions:

- Mix together the diced cucumber and avocado with the lemon juice.
- Flake the tuna and mix well with the mayo and mustard.
- Add the tuna to the avocado and cucumber. Add salt to taste.
- Prepare the salad greens (optional: add olive oil and lemon juice to taste).
- Place the tuna salad on top of the salad greens.
- Sprinkle black pepper on top.

Nutritional Values per serving:

- Calories: 480 Kcal
- Sugar: 2g
- Fat: 40g
- Carbohydrates: 11g
- Fiber: 8g
- Protein: 45g

- **4. Paleo Pressure Cooker Beef And Broccoli**

Prep Time: 5 Minutes

Cook Time: 15 Minutes

Servings: 2

Ingredients:

- 1 tablespoon (15 ml) of olive oil
- 14 oz (400 g) of beef sirloin, cut into bite-size pieces
- 1 teaspoon (2 g) of ginger paste (or minced fresh ginger)
- 1 teaspoon (2 g) of garlic paste (or 1 minced garlic clove)
- 1/2 cup (120 ml) of beef broth
- 1 1/2 tablespoons (23 ml) of gluten-free tamari sauce (or coconut aminos)
- 1/2 head (8 oz or 225 g) of broccoli, broken into small florets
- 1 teaspoon (5 ml) of honey
- Salt and pepper, to taste

Instructions:

- Add the olive oil and beef to the pressure cooker and sauté until browned. Add the ginger paste and garlic paste and sauté for a few seconds. Add the beef broth, tamari sauce, and broccoli to the pressure cooker, stirring to combine.
- Secure the lid on the pressure cooker to close. Set the pressure cooker to cook for 10 minutes and then let the pressure release naturally before removing the lid carefully.
- Remove the beef and broccoli from the pressure cooker with a slotted spoon and set aside to keep warm. To create a sauce, add the honey to the pressure cooker and reduce the liquid by half. Season with salt and pepper, to taste.
- To serve, place the beef and broccoli on 2 plates and spoon equal amounts of the sauce over each plate.

Nutritional Values per serving:

- Calories: 643 Kcal
- Sugar: 4g
- Fat: 49g
- Carbohydrates: 10g
- Fiber: 4g
- Protein: 37g

5. Keto Cottage Pie

Prep Time: 15 Minutes

Cook Time: 1 Hour

Servings: 10

Ingredients:

Base:

- 3 tablespoons olive oil
- 2 cloves garlic crushed
- 1 tablespoon dried oregano
- 1 small onion diced
- 3 sticks celery diced
- 1 teaspoon salt
- 2 pounds ground beef
- 3 tablespoons tomato paste
- 1 cup beef stock
- 1/4 cup red wine vinegar
- 2 tablespoons fresh thyme leaves

10 ounces green beans, cut into 1in lengths *Topping:*

- 1.6 pounds cauliflower cut into florets
- 3 ounces butter
- 1/2 teaspoon salt
- 1/4 teaspoon pepper
- 3 egg yolks
- Pinch paprika
- Pinch dried oregano

Instructions:

Base:

- Place a large saucepan over a high heat.
- Add the olive oil, garlic, oregano, onion and celery and Sauté for 5 minutes, until the onion is starting to become translucent.
- Add the salt and ground beef, stirring continuously to break apart the meat while it browns.
- When the beef is browned add the tomato paste and stir well. Add the
- beef stock and red wine vinegar and simmer uncovered for 20 minutes until the liquid has reduced.
- Add the thyme and green beans and simmer for 5 minutes before removing from the heat.
- Spoon the beef mixture into your casserole dish and set aside.
- Preheat your oven to 175C/350F.

Topping:

- Fill a large saucepan two-thirds full of water and bring to the boil.
- Add the cauliflower and cook for 7-10 minutes until tender.
- Carefully pour the water and cauliflower into a colander and drain well.
- Return the drained cauliflower to the saucepan, along with the butter, salt and pepper.
- Using your stick blender, blend the cauliflower into a smooth mash.
- Add the egg yolks and blend well.
-

Gently spoon the mashed cauliflower onto the beef mixture in your casserole dish.

- Sprinkle with paprika and oregano.
- Bake the pie in the oven for 25-30 minutes, until the mash is golden brown.
- Serve immediately or chill and store in the fridge for up to 1 week.

Nutritional Values per serving:

Serving Size: 210g

- Calories: 420 Kcal
- Carbohydrates: 8g

- Protein: 18g
- Fat: 36g
- Fiber: 4g

6. Paleo Spanish Omelette

Prep Time: 15 minutes

Cook Time: 30 minutes

Servings: 4

Ingredients:

- 3 tablespoons of olive oil (45 ml), to cook with
- 2 medium bell peppers (240 g), diced
- 1 medium onion (110 g), diced
- 1/2 head of cauliflower (300 g), chopped
- 8 medium eggs, whisked
- 1/4 cup (60 ml) coconut cream
- 4 tablespoons (4 g) parsley, choppedSalt and
- pepper, to taste *Instructions:*

- Preheat oven to 350 F (175 C).
- Sauté the bell pepper and onion with the olive oil. Season with salt and pepper to taste. Parboil the cauliflower florets – boil for 2 minutes and drain immediately.
- Mix the eggs, bell pepper, onion, cauliflower, coconut cream, and parsley together in a mixing bowl.
- Pour the mixture into a greased 9-inch by 9-inch (23-cm by 23-cm) square baking dish.
- Make sure to spread the vegetables (especially the cauliflower) out carefully.
- Bake for 20 minutes until the eggs are soft but set.

Nutritional Values per serving:

- Calories: 286 Kcal
- Sugar: 5g
- Fat: 22g
- Carbohydrates: 10g
- Fiber: 3g
- Protein: 14g

7. Simple Paleo Egg Salad

Prep Time: 5 Minutes

Cook Time: 15 Minutes

Servings: 2

Ingredients:

- 4 hard boiled eggs, peeled
- 1/2 tablespoon mustard (add more to taste)
- 1/2 tablespoon mayo (optional – see here for a recipe or here to buy this Paleo mayo online)
- [Optional] 1 tablespoon pickles,
- chopped Salt to taste *Instructions:*

- Cut up the hard boiled eggs into small pieces.
- In a bowl, combine with the mustard, mayo, and salt. Mix well.

Nutritional Values per serving:

- Calories: 268 Kcal
- Fat: 16g
- Carbohydrates: 6g
- Fiber: 1g
- Protein: 22g

8. Pan-Fried Tuscan Chicken Pasta

Prep Time: 10 Minutes

Cook Time: 10 Minutes

Servings: 2

Ingredients:

- 2 chicken breasts, diced
- 2 small egg, whisked
- 1/4 teaspoon salt
- Dash of black pepper
- 2 teaspoons garlic powder
- 2 teaspoons Italian seasoning
- 14 cherry tomatoes, cut into quarters
- 30 basil leaves
- Olive oil or avocado oil to cook in
- Additional salt and pepper to taste

1 zucchini, peeled and turned into shreds or strands for the pasta

Instructions:

- In a bowl, mix together the whisked egg, salt, pepper, garlic powder, and Italian seasoning.
- Place the diced chicken pieces into the egg mixture and make sure the chicken is well covered with the mixture.
- Place 2 tablespoons of olive or avocado oil into a frying pan and sauté the chicken pieces coated with the egg mixture until the chicken pieces are fully cooked.
- Add in the quartered cherry tomatoes and fresh basil leaves. Sauté for 2-3 minutes more.
- Make the zucchini noodles by peeling a zucchini and then using the shredding attachment of a food processor or else using a potato peeler to create pasta-like strands or shreds.
- Divide the zucchini noodles into two and place onto plates. Top with the sautéed chicken.

- *Nutritional Values per serving:*
-
- Calories: 540 Kcal
- Sugar: 4g
- Fat: 36g
  Carbohydrates: 7g
  Fiber: 2g
- Protein: 45g

9. Garlic Shrimp Caesar Salad

Prep Time: 15 Minutes

Cook Time: 10 Minutes

Servings: 4

Ingredients:

For the shrimp:

- 1 lb shrimp (shells removed)
- 2 tablespoons olive oil
- 1 tablespoon lemon juice
- 3 tablespoons garlic powder
- 1 tablespoon onion
-

powder Salt and pepper *For the*

salad:

- 1 head romaine lettuce, chopped
- 1 cucumber, chopped into cubes

For the dressing:

- 1 teaspoon Dijon mustard
- 1/4 cup Paleo mayo (you can purchase this one or make this one)
- 1 tablespoon fresh lemon juice
- 2 teaspoons garlic powder
- Salt and pepper

For garnish:

- 1 tablespoon parsley, chopped – for garnish
- 1 tablespoon sliced almonds – for garnish

Instructions:

- Preheat oven to 400F.
- Mix the shrimp, olive oil, lemon juice, garlic, onion powder, salt and pepper together. Place shrimp on baking tray and roast for 10 minutes.
- To make the salad dressing, blend the mayo, mustard, lemon juice, garlic powder, salt and pepper together.
- Toss the dressing with the chopped lettuce, chopped cucumber, and roasted shrimp. Garnish with the chopped parsley and sliced almonds.

Nutritional Values per serving:

Serving Size: 330 g

- Calories: 296 Kcal
- Sugar: 2g
- Fat: 19g
- Carbohydrates: 7g
- Fiber: 4g
- Protein: 25g

10. Zucchini noodles with avocado sauce

Prep time: 10 mins

Servings: 2

- These delicious zucchini noodles (or zoodles) with avocado sauce are
- ready in 10 minutes. Besides, this recipe requires just 7 ingredients to
- make.
-
- *Ingredients:*

- 1 zucchini
- 1 1/4 cup basil (30 g)

1/3 cup water (85 ml)
4 tbsp pine nuts
2 tablespoons lemon juice
1 avocado
12 sliced cherry tomatoes

Instructions:

- Make the zucchini noodles using a peeler or the Spiralizer. Blend
- the rest of the ingredients (except the cherry tomatoes) in a blender until smooth.
- Combine noodles, avocado sauce and cherry tomatoes in a mixing bowl.
- These zucchini noodles with avocado sauce are better fresh, but you can store them in the fridge for 1 to 2 days.

Recipe Notes:

Feel free to use any veggies or fresh herbs you have on hand. You can also spiralize other veggies like carrots, beet, butternut squash, cabbage, etc.

Any nuts can be used instead of the pine nuts, or even seeds.

Nutritional Values per serving:

- Calories: 313 Kcal
- Sugar: 6.5g
- Fat: 26.8g
- Carbohydrates: 18.7g
- Fiber: 9.7g
- Protein: 6.8g

11. Paleo Chicken Noodle Soup Recipe

Prep Time: 15 Minutes

Cook Time: 15 Minutes

Yield: 2 bowls

Ingredients:

- 3 cups chicken broth (use this recipe or buy this one) (approx 720ml)
- 1 chicken breast, chopped into small pieces (approx 240g or 0.5
- lb)
- 2 tablespoons avocado oil
- 1 stalk of celery, chopped (approx 57g)
- 1 green onion, chopped (approx 10g)
- 1/4 cup cilantro, finely chopped (approx 15g)
- 1 zucchini, peeled (approx

106g) Salt to taste *Instructions:*

- Dice the chicken breast.
- Add the avocado oil into a saucepan and sauté the diced chicken in there until cooked.
- Add chicken broth to the same saucepan and simmer.
- Chop the celery and add it into the saucepan.
- Chop the green onions and add them into the saucepan.
- Chop the cilantro and put it aside for the moment.
-

- Create zucchini noodles – I used a potato peeler to create long strands,
- but other options include using a spiralizer or a food processor with the
- shredding attachment.
- Add zucchini noodles and cilantro to the pot.
- Simmer for a few more minutes, add salt to taste, and serve immediately.

Nutritional Values per serving (1 bowl):

- Calories: 310 Kcal
- Sugar: 3g
- Fat: 16g
- Carbohydrates: 6g
- Fiber: 2g
- Protein: 34g

12. Keto Beef Teriyaki Recipe with Sesame and Kale

Prep Time: 10 Minutes

Cook Time: 10 Minutes

Servings: 2

Ingredients:

- 2 tablespoons of gluten-free tamari sauce or coconut aminos (30 ml)
- 1 tablespoon of applesauce (15 ml)
- 2 cloves of garlic (6 g), minced
- 1 tablespoon of fresh ginger (4 g), minced
- 2 beef sirloin steaks (400 g) (pick a well marbled steak), sliced
- 1 tablespoon of sesame seeds (14 g)
- 1 teaspoon of sesame oil (5 ml)
- 2 tablespoons of avocado oil (30 ml)
- 10 white button mushrooms (100 g), sliced
- 2 oz of curly kale (56 g) Salt and pepper, to

taste *Instructions:*

- Whisk the tamari sauce, applesauce, garlic and ginger together in a bowl. Add the sliced sirloin and leave to marinate while you prep the remaining ingredients.
- Toast the sesame seeds in a hot, dry pan until golden. Remove and set aside.
- Heat the avocado oil in a large wok or frying pan and add the mushrooms, cooking until caramelised. Add the steak slices and the marinade and fry for 2-3 minutes, adding the kale towards the end, stirring into the mixture to gently wilt.
- Add in the sesame oil and salt and pepper to taste.
- Serve over cooked cauliflower rice if desired, and top with toasted sesame seeds.

Nutritional Values per serving:

- Calories: 675 Kcal

- Sugar: 2g
- Fat: 53g
- Carbohydrates: 9g
- Fiber: 3g
- Protein: 38g

13. Keto Turkey and Vegetable Skillet

Prep Time: 10 Minutes

Cook Time: 15 Minutes

Servings: 2

Ingredients:

- 3 tablespoons of coconut oil (90 ml), to cook with
- 0.75 lb of turkey breasts (335 g), diced (or ground turkey)
- 4 slices of bacon (112 g), diced
- 1/2 medium onion (55 g), diced
- 3 spears of asparagus (45 g), chopped
- 1 cup of spinach (30 g), chopped
- 4 teaspoons of fresh thyme (4 g),

chopped Salt and pepper, to taste *Instructions:*

- In a large skillet, melt the coconut oil over medium-high heat. Add the turkey and bacon to the skillet and sauté until slightly browned about 5 to 7 minutes.
- Add the onion, asparagus, spinach and fresh thyme to the skillet. Sauté for an additional 10 minutes until the turkey and bacon are cooked through and the vegetables are soft.
- Season with salt and pepper, to taste.

Nutritional Values per serving:

- Calories: 665 Kcal

- Sugar: 2g
- Fat: 52g
- Carbohydrates: 5g
  Fiber: 2g
- Protein: 47g

14. Vegan thai soup

Prep time: 10 Minutes

Cook time: 15 Minutes

Servings: 3-4

You only need one pot to make this delicious vegan Thai soup. It's made with easy to get ingredients and you can add your favorite veggies.

Ingredients:

- 1/2 julienned red onion
- 1/2 julienned red bell pepper
- 3 sliced mushrooms
- 2 cloves of garlic, finely chopped
- 1/2-inch piece of ginger root (about 1 cm), peeled and finely chopped
- 1/2 Thai chili, finely chopped*
- 2 cups vegetable broth or water (500 ml)
- 1 14-ounce can coconut milk (400 ml)
- 1 tablespoon coconut, cane or brown sugar
- 10 oz firm tofu, cubed (275 g)
- 1 tbsp tamari or soy sauce
- The juice of half a lime

A handful of fresh cilantro, chopped *Instructions:*

- Place all the veggies (onion, red bell pepper, mushrooms, garlic, ginger and Thai chili), broth, coconut milk and sugar in a large pot.
  Bring it to a boil and then cook over medium heat for about 5 minutes.

-
-

- Add the tofu and cook for 5 minutes more.
  Remove from the heat, add the tamari, lime juice and fresh cilantro.
  Stir and serve.
  Keep the soup in a sealed container in the fridge for up to 5 days. You can also freeze it.

Notes:

* Feel free to use any type of chili you want.

Nutritional Values per serving:

- Calories: 339 Kcal
- Sugar: 5.3g
- Fat: 27.6g
- Carbohydrates: 15.6g
- Fiber: 3.2g
- Protein: 14.8g

15. Vegan Cauliflower Fried Rice

Prep Time: 10 Minutes

Cook Time: 15 Minutes

Servings: 3

Ingredients:

-
-

- 1/2 teaspoon oil (optional)
- 1/4 cup (40 g) onion or shallots, chopped
- 4 cloves of garlic finely chopped
- 1 tablespoon minced ginger
- 1 cup (140 g) peas and carrots
- 1/2 cup (74.5 g) chopped bell pepper
- 1/2 (0.5) head of medium cauliflower, 2.5 to 3 cups shredded
- 1/4 (0.25) head of broccoli, about 1 cup shredded, or use more cauliflower

1 tablespoon + 1 tsp soy sauce
1 to 2 tsp sambal oelek or asian chile sauce

- 1/2 to 1 tsp toasted sesame oil

1/4 teaspoon (0.25 tsp) salt

- A generous dash of black
- pepper Scallions for garnish

Instructions:

- Cook onion and garlic in oil (or 1 tbsp broth) over medium heat until golden. Add ginger, bell pepper, veggies, peas and carrots and a dash of salt. Mix, cover and cook for 3 to 4 minutes.
- Add the shredded cauliflower or cauliflower+ broccoli, sauces, salt and pepper and mix well.
- Cover and cook for 5 minutes. Fluff really well, cover and let sit to steam for another 2 minutes. You want the cauliflower to be cooked to a bit more than al dente, but still have just a slight bite.
- Taste and adjust salt, flavor. Fluff again. Serve hot as is or with some stir fry or baked tofu. Add some asian chile sauce or some soy sauce for garnish when serving as is. You can serve it with some stir fry like the Baked Tofu and Eggplant with Soy Lime Sauce.

Notes:

-
-

- To add egg sub: Crumble up 1/4 cup tofu and add to the pan at step 1 after the onions have cooked. Cook until heated through, add a good pinch of turmeric and Indian black salt (kala namak) and mix. Continue adding the ginger and veggies.

Add some toasted nuts with the cauliflower for variation.

Use coconut aminos to make soy-free.

Nutritional Values per serving:

- Calories: 106 Kcal
- Fat: 3g
  Carbohydrates: 17g

  Fiber: 5g
  Protein: 5g

16. Easy Keto Chili

Prep time: 10 Minutes

Cook time: 30 Minutes

Servings: 6

Ingredients:

-

-
-

- 1 pound of lean ground beef
- 2 cloves garlic crushed
- 1 tablespoon olive oil
- 1 medium onion roughly chopped
- 28 oz can crushed tomato
- 1 cup of chopped cherry tomatoes
- 1 cup of water
- 1 ½ teaspoons of sea salt
- 2 tablespoons of chili powder
- ½ tsp ground cayenne pepper
- 1 tablespoon of cumin powder
- 1 teaspoon of garlic powder

2 teaspoons of onion powder*Instructions:*

- Brown the ground beef, onions, garlic
- Add the can of tomatoes, fresh tomatoes, water, and spices.
- Allow to simmer on medium low heat for 30-45 minutes.
- Alternatively you can cook this chili in slow cooker to do so refer to the notes section.
- This recipe double and freezes well.

Recipe Notes:

Slow Cooker Instructions:

- Add all the ingredients into your slow cooker and break up the ground beef and then set to low. Your Keto Chili will be done in 4-6 hours, based on your specific slow cooker.

Nutritional Values per serving:

- Calories: 178 Kcal
- Fat: 5.5g
- Carbohtydrates: 7.3g
- Fiber: 2.2g
- Sugar: 2.2g
- Protein: 24.3g

17.Keto Air Fryer Fish Sticks

Prep Time: 10 Minutes

Cook Time: 10 Minutes

Servings: 4

Ingredients:

- 1 lb white fish such as cod
- 1/4 cup mayonnaise
- 2 tablespoons Dijon mustard
- 2 tbsp water
- 1 1/2 cups pork rind panko such as Pork King Good
- 3/4 tsp cajun seasoning
- Salt and pepper to taste

Instructions:

- Spray the air fryer rack with non-stick cooking spray (I use avocado oil spray).

- Pat the fish dry and cut into sticks about 1 inch by 2 inches wide (how you are able to cut it will depend a little on what kind of fish you buy and how thick and wide it is).
- In a small shallow bowl, whisk together the mayo, mustard, and water. In another shallow bowl, whisk together the pork rinds and Cajun seasoning. Add salt and pepper to taste (both the pork rinds and seasoning could have a fair bit of salt, so dip a finger in to taste how salty it is).
- Working with one piece of fish at a time, dip into the mayo mixture to coat and then tap off the excess. Dip into the pork rind mixture and toss to coat. Place on the air fryer rack.
- Set to Air Fry at 400F and bake 5 minutes, the flip the fish sticks with tongs and bake another 5 minutes. Serve immediately.

Recipe Notes:

If you don't have an air fryer, you can still make these delicious keto fish sticks. Simply preheat your oven to 425F and add several tablespoons of oil to a rimmed sheet pan. Place the sheet pan in the oven while it preheats. Place the coated fish sticks on the pan and bake 5 minutes, then flip over and bake another 5 minutes.

Nutritional Values per serving :

- Fat: 16g
- Carbohydrates: 1g
- Fiber: 0.5g
- Protein: 26.4g
- Calories: 263 kcal

18. Keto zuppa toscana

Prep Time: 10 Minutes

Cook Time: 45 Minutes

Servings: 8

Ingredients:

- 6 slices bacon, roughly chopped
- 1 lb ground mild Italian sausage
- 1 tbsp (14g) butter
- 2 tsp (10g) minced garlic
- ½ tsp ground sage
- ¼ tsp black pepper
- 2 ¾ cups chicken broth
- ¾ cup heavy whipping cream
- ¼ cup shredded parmesan cheese
- 1 lb radishes, quartered
- 2 oz kale, de-stemmed, roughly chopped

Instructions:

- To a large pot over medium heat, cook chopped bacon until crisp. Transfer bacon to a paper-towel-lined plate and dispose of grease, but do not wash the pan.
- In the same pot over medium-high heat, cook ground sausage until browned, breaking the meat apart with a wooden spoon while cooking. Transfer browned sausage to a paper towel-lined plate and dispose of grease, but do not wash the pan.
- To same pot over medium heat, melt butter. Add garlic and spices and sauté until fragrant, about 1 minute. Increase heat to medium-high and add in chicken broth, heavy cream, and shredded parmesan. Bring mixture to a simmer, add quartered radishes, and decrease the heat to medium-low. Simmer until radishes are fork-tender, about 15-20 minutes.
- Stir in browned sausage and chopped kale and continue to simmer until kale wilts, about 5-10 minutes, before serving in bowls. Garnish soup with crisped bacon crumbles.

Nutritional Values per serving:

- Calories: 334 Kcal
- Fat: 31g
- Carbohydrates: 3.9g
- Dietary Fiber: 1.1g
- Protein: 12g

19. Taco Casseroele - Low Carb/Keto

Prep time: 20 Minutes

Cook time: 20 Minutes

Servings: 6

Ingredients:

- 1 1/2 lb ground beef
- 1 14.5 oz can chopped tomatoes
- 1 4 oz can diced green chiles
- 2 cups cooked cauliflower rice
- 3 tbs taco seasoning
- 1 8 oz bag taco cheese

Instructions:

- Cook the cauliflower rice (either bagged or fresh) and pat dry to remove excess moisture.
- Cook beef on stovetop until brown.
- Add tomatoes, cauliflower, taco seasoning and chiles and stir until well mixed.
- In a 13 x 9 baking dish, layer enough of the beef mixture to cover the bottom - about half.
- Top with 2/3 of the cheese and spread evenly.
- Repeat with the rest of the beef and then top with the rest of the cheese.
- Bake for 15-20 min at 350 degrees until cheese is melted.
- Serve in a bowl alone or with sour cream and avocado.

Nutritional Values per serving:

- Calories: 522 Kcal
- Fat: 31g
- Carbohydrates: 10g
- Fiber: 3g
- Protein: 42g

20. Broccoli Bacon Salad with Onions and Coconut Cream

Prep Time: 10 Minutes

Cook Time: 30 Minutes

Servings: 6

Ingredients:

- 1 lb broccoli florets
- 4 small red onions or 2 large ones, sliced
- 20 slices of bacon, chopped into small pieces
- 1 cup coconut cream
- Salt to taste

Instructions:

- Cook the bacon first, and then cook the onions in the bacon fat.
- Blanche the broccoli florets (or you can use them raw or have them softer by boiling them).
- Toss the bacon pieces, onions, and broccoli florets together with the coconut cream and salt to taste.
- Serve at room temperature.

Nutritional Values per serving:

Serving Size: 1 bowl

- Calories: 280 Kcal
- Sugar: 2g
- Fat: 26g
- Carbohydrates: 8g
- Fiber: 3g
- Protein: 7g

21. Keto Chicken Mushroom Casserole

Prep Time: 10 Minutes

Cook Time: 40 Minutes

Servings: 4

Ingredients:

- 4 tablespoons of avocado oil (30 ml), to cook with
- 8 chicken thighs (with skin on) (1.2 kg)
- 1 medium onion (110 g), peeled and thinly sliced
- 3 cloves of garlic (9 g), peeled and chopped
- 2 tablespoons of fresh rosemary (6 g), chopped
- 30 white button mushrooms (300 g), halved
- 2 oz of kale (56 g)
- Salt and freshly ground black pepper
- Additional rosemary sprigs for garnish (optional)

Instructions:

- Preheat the oven to 350°F (180°C).
- Add avocado oil to a frying pan and brown the chicken thighs skinside down until golden and crispy, then turn the thighs over and cook the other side for a minute or two.
- The chicken isn't cooked right now, but will be finished off in the oven. Carefully remove from the frying pan and put into a roasting dish.
- Using the leftover oil in the pan, cook the sliced onions, garlic and rosemary and cook over a low-moderate heat to soften the onions

completely. Turn the heat up and keep cooking the onions for a few more minutes until they become jammy. Add the mushrooms to the frying pan for a few minutes.

- Spoon the mushrooms and jammy onions into the roasting tray around the chicken pieces and place the dish in the oven for 20 minutes.
- In the meantime, toss the kale in some more olive oil.
- After 20 minutes, increase the oven temperature to 400 F (200 C) and remove the tray from the oven while it heats. Scatter the oiled kale in and around the dish, then return the dish to the oven for an additional 5 minutes.
- Season with salt and freshly ground black pepper, as well as additional rosemary sprigs, then serve to the table for everyone to help themselves.

Nutritional Values per serving:

- Calories: 553 Kcal
- Sugar: 3g
- Fat: 42g
- Carbohydrates: 7g
- Fiber: 2g
- Protein: 35g

22. 3-Ingredient Creamy Keto Salmon "Pasta" Recipe

Prep Time: 5 Minutes

Cook Time: 5 Minutes

Servings: 2

Ingredients:

- 2 tablespoons of coconut oil (30 ml), to cook with
- 8 oz of smoked salmon (224 g), diced
- 2 zucchinis (240 g), spiraled or use a peeler to make into long noodlelike strands

- 1/4 cup of mayo (60 ml) *Instructions:*

- In a skillet, melt the coconut oil over medium-high heat. Add the smoked salmon and sauté until slightly browned, about 2 to 3 minutes. • Add the zucchini "noodles" to the skillet and sauté until soft, about 1 to 2 minutes.
- Add the mayo to the skillet, stirring well to combine.

- Divide the "pasta" between 2 plates and serve.

Nutritional Values per serving:

- Calories: 470 Kcal
- Sugar: 2g
- Fat: 42g
- Carbohydrates: 4g
- Fiber: 1g
- Protein: 21g

23. Mini Spinach Meatloaves

Prep Time: 5 Minutes

Cook Time: 20 Minutes

Yield: 12 Muffins

Ingredients:

- 1/4 lb (113 g) ground pork or ground turkey
- 1/4 lb(113 g) ground beef
- 1/2 small onion (55 g), diced
- 2 cloves garlic, minced
- 1/3 lb (140 g) fresh spinach, chopped small
- 4 eggs, whisked
- 2 tablespoons Italian seasoning
- 1/2 tablespoon salt
- 1/2 teaspoon black pepper
- 1/3 cup (80 ml) almond or coconut

milk Coconut oil to sauté in *Instructions:*

- Preheat oven to 400 F (200 C).
- Saute the meat, diced onions, and garlic in 1 tablespoon of coconut oil. When the meat is cooked, add in the chopped spinach and sauté for 1-2 minutes longer.
- Place muffin cup liners into a 12-cup muffin pan.
- In a large bowl, combine the sauté with the whisked eggs, Italian seasoning, salt, black pepper, and almond or coconut milk.
- Divide the mixture between the 12 muffin cups.
- Bake for 10 minutes until each muffin is pretty solid. Cook for longer if the muffins are still liquidy.

Nutritional Values per serving:

Serving Size: 6 muffins

- Calories: 430 Kcal
- Sugar: 2g
- Fat: 30g
- Carbohydrates: 7g
- Fiber: 3g
- Protein: 30g

24. Cobb Egg Salad

Prep Time: 15 Minutes

Cook Time: 10 Minutes

Servings: 4

Ingredients:

- 3 tablespoons nonfat plain yogurt
- 3 tablespoons low-fat mayonnaise
- ¼ teaspoon garlic powder
- ¼ teaspoon freshly ground pepper
- ⅛ teaspoon salt
- 8 hard-boiled eggs (see Tip)
- 1 ripe avocado, cubed
- 2 slices bacon, cooked and crumbled
- ¼ cup crumbled blue cheese

Instructions:

- Combine yogurt, mayonnaise, garlic powder, pepper and salt in a medium bowl.
- Halve eggs and discard 4 of the yolks (or save for another use). Add
- whites and the remaining 4 yolks to the bowl and mash to desired consistency.
- Gently stir in avocado, bacon and blue cheese.

Make Ahead Tip: Cover and refrigerate for up to 2 days.

Tip : To hard-boil eggs, place eggs in a single layer in a saucepan; cover with water. Bring to a simmer over medium-high heat. Reduce heat to low and cook at the barest simmer for 10 minutes. Remove from heat, pour out hot water and cover the eggs with ice-cold water. Let stand until cool enough to handle before peeling.

Nutritional Values per serving:

Serving size: about ¾ cup

- Calories: 235 Kcal
- Fat: 17g
- Fiber: 3g
- Carbohydrates: 9g
- Protein: 3g

CONCLUSION

Intermittent fasting isn't starving yourself to lose weight right. Intermittent fasting isn't a diet. It's a pattern of eating. To be more exact, it's a lifestyle to carry on for life.

And as a lifestyle, it's very important to track and measure your progress.

In conclusion, intermittent fasting is one of the simplest and most effective methods you have to improve your overall wellbeing and is a great tool for weight management.

THE WARRIOR DIET

	DAY 1	DAY 2	DAY 3	DAY 4	DAY 5	DAY 6	DAY 7
Midnight 4 AM 8 AM 12 PM	Eating only small amounts of vegetables and fruits	Eating only small amounts of vegetables and fruits	Eating only small amounts of vegetables and fruits	Eating only small amounts of vegetables and fruits	Eating only small amounts of vegetables and fruits	Eating only small amounts of vegetables and fruits	Eating only small amounts of vegetables and fruits
4 PM	Large meal	Large meal	Large meal	Large meal	Large meal	Large meal	Large meal
8 PM Midnight							

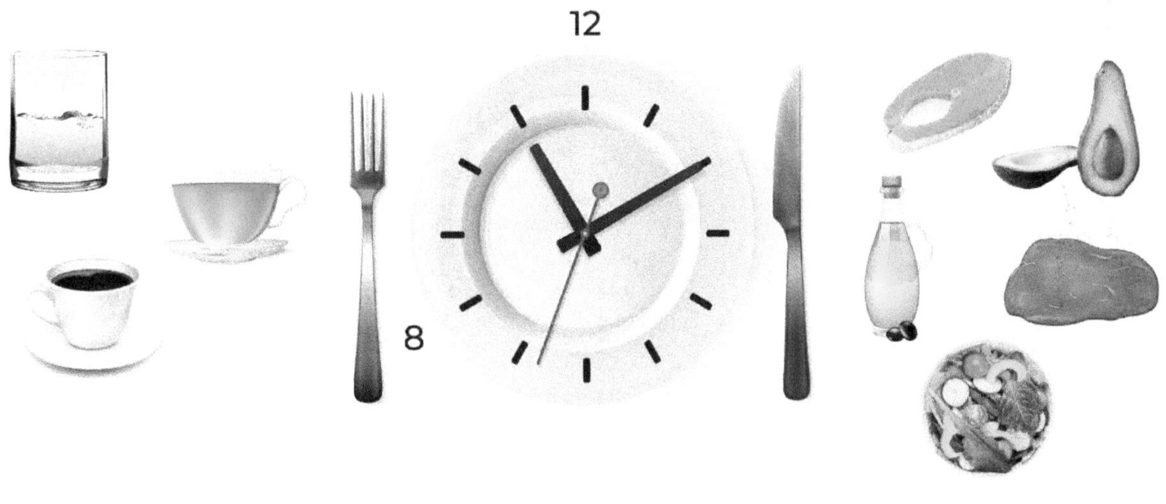
12
8

CPSIA information can be obtained
at www.ICGtesting.com
Printed in the USA
BVHW092107180821
614616BV00016B/945

9 781915 032584